Disulfiram

Avinash De Sousa

Disulfiram

Its Use in Alcohol Dependence and Other Disorders

Springer

Avinash De Sousa
Department of Psychiatry
Lokmanya Tilak Muncipal Medical College
Mumbai
India

ISBN 978-981-32-9875-0 ISBN 978-981-32-9876-7 (eBook)
https://doi.org/10.1007/978-981-32-9876-7

This Springer imprint is published by the registered company Springer Nature Singapore Pte Ltd.
The registered company address is: 152 Beach Road, #21-01/04 Gateway East, Singapore 189721, Singapore

Preface

This is a unique and one of its kind book dedicated to a drug named Disulfiram, which has been used in the management of alcohol dependence for the past six decades. The book has eight chapters and traces the history of evolution of Disulfiram, its mechanism of action, its role in alcohol and cocaine dependence, its side effects and toxicity, its use in special populations and its future with certain ethical issues. The book will serve to help clinicians and students alike in understanding various facets of Disulfiram and its usage.

This book is dedicated to my late father Prof. Dr. Alan De Sousa who introduced me to Disulfiram and with whom my early work in Disulfiram is associated.

I am sure readers will enjoy reading the book as much I have enjoyed writing it.

Mumbai, India

Avinash De Sousa

Contents

1 Disulfiram: The History Behind the Molecule 1
1.1 Introduction 1
1.2 Early History of Disulfiram 2
1.3 Disulfiram as a Pharmacological Agent. 2
1.4 Disulfiram and the Name 'Antabuse'. 3
1.5 Early Historical Clinical Disulfiram Research. 4
1.6 Early Disulfiram and Ethanol Metabolism Research. 5
1.7 Further Usage of Disulfiram in the Early Period 6
1.8 Discovery of the Non-Alcohol Uses of Disulfiram 6
References. 6

2 Disulfiram: Pharmacology and Mechanism of Action. 9
2.1 Introduction 9
2.2 Mechanism of Action of Disulfiram 9
2.3 Disulfiram Metabolism in Human Subjects. 10
2.4 Disulfiram and Its Action via Dopamine 11
2.5 Absorption and Biotransformation of Disulfiram 12
2.6 Distribution and Excretion of Disulfiram. 13
2.7 Aldehyde Dehydrogenase Enzymes 13
2.8 Pharmacokinetics of Disulfiram. 14
2.9 Measuring Compliance When on Disulfiram Therapy 14
2.10 Drug Interactions with Disulfiram. 15
2.11 Conclusion 16
References. 16

3 Disulfiram in the Management of Alcohol Dependence 21
3.1 Introduction 21
3.2 Studies of Disulfiram in Patients with Alcohol Dependence. 22
3.3 Disulfiram Implant Therapy. 26
3.4 Do Certain Patients Respond Better to Disulfiram Therapy? 27
3.5 Points of Clinical Relevance 27
3.6 Conclusion 28
References. 28

4 **Disulfiram in the Management of Cocaine Dependence and Other Psychiatric Disorders** 31
4.1 Introduction 31
4.2 Mechanism of Action of Disulfiram in Cocaine Dependence 31
4.3 Disulfiram in Cocaine Dependence—A Review of Studies Done 32
4.4 Some Other Hypotheses on the Mechanism of Action of Disulfiram in Cocaine Dependence 36
4.5 Disulfiram and Its Potential Role in the Management of Pathological Gambling 37
4.6 Some Points of Clinical Relevance 38
4.7 Conclusion 39
References 39

5 **Disulfiram in Comparison and Combination with Other Agents in the Management of Alcohol Dependence** 43
5.1 Introduction 43
5.2 Disulfiram in Comparison with Other Agents in Alcohol Dependence 43
5.3 Disulfiram Combined with Other Agents in the Alcohol Dependence 45
5.4 Combining Disulfiram with Other Drugs—A Clinical Approach 46
5.5 Disulfiram and Naltrexone 46
5.6 Disulfiram and Acamprosate 47
5.7 Disulfiram and Topiramate 47
5.8 Disulfiram and Baclofen 48
5.9 Conclusion 48
References 49

6 **Disulfiram and Its Use in Special Populations** 51
6.1 Introduction 51
6.2 Disulfiram in the Elderly 51
6.3 Disulfiram Use in Adolescents 52
6.4 Disulfiram in Female Patients and Pregnancy 53
6.5 Disulfiram Use in Patients with Dual Diagnosis 54
6.6 Disulfiram Use in Opioid-Dependent Populations 55
6.7 Disulfiram in Binge Eating Disorder 55
6.8 Positron Emission Tomography Studies with Disulfiram 55
6.9 Conclusion 56
References 56

7 **Disulfiram: Side Effects and Toxicity** 59
7.1 Introduction 59
7.2 Liver Toxicity 59
7.3 Neuropathy 60
7.4 Psychosis 61
7.5 Catatonia 61

7.6 Other Side Effects 62
7.7 Disulfiram–Ethanol Reactions 63
7.8 Disulfiram-Induced Skin Reactions 64
7.9 Mortality with Disulfiram 64
7.10 Conclusion 64
References 64

8 Disulfiram: Clinical Pearls, Ethics and Future Needs 69
8.1 Introduction 69
8.2 Clinical Pearls on Disulfiram 69
8.3 Surreptitious Use of Disulfiram 72
8.4 Why Is Disulfiram Under-Prescribed and Why Does It Face Opposition 73
8.5 Technique of Effective Supervised Disulfiram Therapy 74
8.6 Conclusions 75
References 76

About the Author

Avinash De Sousa is a Consultant Psychiatrist and Psychotherapist. He currently works as a Research Associate in the Department of Psychiatry at Lokmanya Tilak Municipal Medical College in Mumbai, India. He is also the Founder Trustee of the Desousa Foundation, a trust that works in the area of mental health awareness across all sectors. As a Visiting Faculty Member and Professor, he is frequently engaged in various Teacher Training Courses across Mumbai and across India. He has produced more than 650 publications in national and international journals and is the author of 6 books in the area of mental health. His primary research interests are in child psychiatry, alcohol dependence, Disulfiram and schizophrenia. One of the few psychiatrists who in addition to a psychiatry degree also holds a master's degree in Counseling and Psychotherapy, an M Phil in Applied Psychology and an MBA in Human Resource Development, he was also awarded a Doctorate in Clinical Psychology from the University of Hertfordshire (UK) in 2011.

Disulfiram: The History Behind the Molecule

1

1.1 Introduction

Disulfiram has been used now all over the world in the long-term management of alcohol dependence. Disulfiram or Antabuse®, as it is popularly known abroad, is the pharmacological name for an organic sulphur compound, which is chemically composed of tetraethylthiuram disulfide (disulfiram) which is a light-grey crystalline powder. It possesses a molecular weight of 296.54 [1]. It was over 70 years ago, in 1945 that Danish researchers observed that this substance caused significant unpleasant physiological adverse effects in individuals after the consumption of alcohol. It was only after a few years that this molecule was used in the long-term management of alcohol dependence. The drug was then also being used in Denmark but on a lesser scale internationally. It is interesting that literature is abound with data on Disulfiram and its effects on the long-term management of alcohol dependence both in the form of reviews and clinical trials, while literature on the history and discovery of Disulfiram is scarce [2]. This chapter aims to bridge the gap by providing the reader a detailed account of the history and discovery of Disulfiram as a molecule (Fig. 1.1).

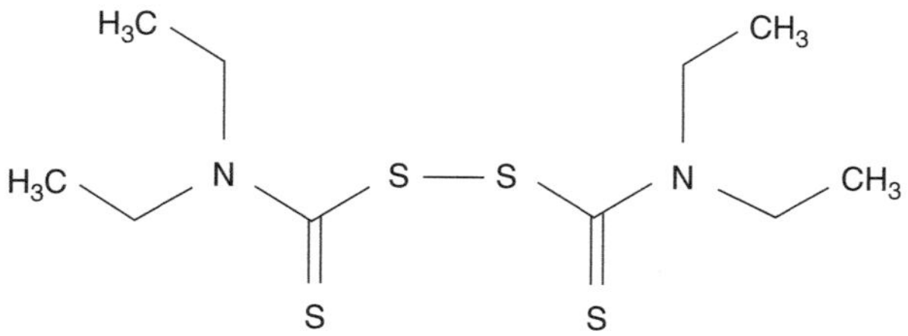

Fig. 1.1 The chemical formula of Disulfiram. (Source—www.caymanchem.com)

A. De Sousa, *Disulfiram*, https://doi.org/10.1007/978-981-32-9876-7_1

1.2 Early History of Disulfiram

The early history shall trace how the effect of disulfiram on ethanol metabolism and its action was discovered, how it came to be marketed as an agent for the treatment of alcohol dependence and the early clinical use of the molecule. It is worthwhile mentioning that the discovery of Disulfiram was by serendipity, which then changed the face of alcohol dependence management for many years to come. While the discovery of disulfiram as a drug has been dated as the late 1940s, the drug has been known in medicine since the late 1800s. A German chemist Grodzki, reported in 1881, about a new compound synthesized from thiocarbamide [3]. He evoked a lukewarm response from the scientific community at that point of time, and it was in an era when organic chemistry was in its heyday and new chemicals were synthesized via various chemical reactions. Two decades after the discovery of this chemical, disulfiram was being used in the rubber industry to facilitate the faster vulcanization of rubber [4]. It was a very useful chemical and was used worldwide in the rubber industry. It was in connection with the rubber industry that disulfiram was first discovered as a deterrent to alcohol use. In 1937, E.E. Williams, a plant physician in the American rubber industry, described in a report that workers in the plant, processing tetramethylthiuram monosulfide and disulfide, suffered a reaction and uneasiness when ingesting alcohol [5]. It was thought that these negative properties of disulfiram might perhaps lead to the cure for alcohol dependence but this was not taken up scientifically or in studies. The effect of disulfiram on alcohol ingestion was also reported in the Swedish rubber industry. However the effects of disulfiram as a drug to manage alcohol was not tried out at that time [6]. It had been known at that time that cyanamides produce hypersensitivity to alcohol in workers in the cyanamide industry. This was described and reported in Germany in 1914, but the causal theories for these mechanisms were undiscovered. At that time the role of cyanamide in the management of alcohol dependence was not studied [7].

1.3 Disulfiram as a Pharmacological Agent

Disulfiram was also used in the 1940s by dermatologists for the treatment of scabies. In 1942 two British physicians concluded that it was indeed a useful drug for the management of scabies. The effect of the disulfide in destroying scabies and intestinal worms was investigated in Sweden in 1943 when disulfiram was used in the management of animals infested with worms and scabies. Pharmacological companies at that time began marketing the drug for animal and human scabies manifestations [8].

In 1934, Erik Jacobsen was the head of a pharmaceutical company and its biomedical research unit in Copenhagen. He was appointed in 1962 as professor of pharmacology at the Pharmaceutical College, an institution established in 1892 and merged with the University of Copenhagen. Jacobsen's research area was problems of cell oxidation, and he discovered that the anti-scabies effect of disulfiram was due to its ability to absorb copper and form chelates with the metal. Animal experiments revealed that the drug would work also for intestinal worms. The experiments confirmed that the drug was a vermicide. Human experimentation for disulfiram as a vermicide was yet to be done [9]. Jacobsen, a pharmacologist at that time, had the habit of ingesting experimental drugs on his own to see their effects. He ingested disulfiram before going for a dinner event as it was known at that time (or thought to be) to be useful in the ablation of intestinal worms. On doing so, he later realized at the dinner that he was unable to tolerate alcohol and even a sip of an alcoholic drink led to flushing in his face, feeling uneasy and breathless. He was thus forced not to drink at the event [10]. There have been accounts where on forcibly drinking alcohol after disulfiram, Jacobsen reported that his blood pressure fell and he felt giddy and as though he would be dead soon [11]. Thus in a few days it was confirmed that disulfiram has adverse effects on human beings when they ingested alcohol.

In 1945, Jacobsen and his collaborators realized that disulfiram had the potential to be used as a drug for long-term treatment of alcohol dependence but they did not follow up the idea. Alcohol dependence at that time was not a public health issue in Denmark, and an alcohol-deterrent drug was of little commercial interest to the pharmaceutical industry [12]. Two years later in 1947, Jacobsen established scientific contact with Oluf Martensen-Larsen, a physician who had experience with treatment of alcohol-dependent patients. They initiated systematic studies in order to develop a disulfiram-based drug, to understand its physiological actions in human subjects and establish its efficacy in clinical trials on alcohol dependence. Experiments confirmed that the disulfiram–ethanol reaction mainly took place in the liver, the most important organ capable of metabolizing alcohol [13]. Jacobsen and his colleague Hald had realized the importance of acetaldehyde in the genesis of the disulfiram–ethanol reaction [14]. According to Jacobsen, he mentions '*One of our collaborators, a chemist, happened to enter the laboratory and pointed out the strong smell of acetaldehyde. We, being present in the room, had not noticed the smell because we had slowly adapted to it. This observation gave us the key to understand the process. Further experiments proved that when acetaldyhyde was injected intravenously it resulted in the same symptoms as previously experienced when ingesting alcohol after consuming disulfiram*' [14]. Enzyme studies had proved that oxidation of acetaldehyde, the first step in the metabolism of ethanol, was impeded by disulfiram in human subjects.

1.4 Disulfiram and the Name 'Antabuse'

An accidental observation paved the way for the naming of disulfiram as 'Antabuse'. A sample of disulfiram was accidentally polluted with small amounts of copper, and Jacobsen and his group noticed that the dark precipitate did not disappear by following the standard procedure of washing with ethanol. They succeeded in removing the precipitate by recrystallizing with carbon tetrachloride and in this way also securing a better drug. Disulfiram in this form was easily absorbed in the organism. This form of disulfiram is named antabuse (or 'antabus' in Danish). This was granted a Danish patent in 1952, with patent protection retroactive from 1949 [15]. This Danish version of the name was also used by English and American companies worldwide.

1.5 Early Historical Clinical Disulfiram Research

The discovery of the effect of disulfiram in preventing intake of alcohol was announced to an international audience in an invited lecture Jacobsen gave to the annual meeting of the British Pharmacological Society in July, 1948. His group later presented many aspects of the disulfiram–ethanol reaction. Their research in 1948–49 was impressive. The early studies were published in *Acta Pharmacologica et Toxicologica*, an international journal founded in 1945 and edited by Scandinavian researchers. The fact that it was published in Copenhagen and that Jacobsen was among the editors made it an ideal journal for publishing new research related to disulfiram. Some journal issues had even 2–3 papers on Disulfiram published by Jacobsen and his group [16].

Hald and Jacobsen in their early experiments measured acetaldehyde in the blood of individuals treated with disulfiram by means of a colour reaction with *p*-hydroxydiphenyl. In order to be certain that the increase found was really due to acetaldehyde, they chemically isolated and identified acetaldehyde in the expired air. They noticed an eight-time increase in acetaldehyde concentration when 40 ml of alcohol was consumed after 1.5 g of disulfiram being taken the previous day [17]. The medical world zoomed in on disulfiram via the papers by Jacobsen and Martensen-Larsen that appeared in *The Lancet* in December, 1948. The paper read "*Alcohol given to persons previously treated with this otherwise innocuous substance produces dilatation of the facial vessels, increased pulmonary ventilation, raised pulse-rate, and general uneasiness. The symptoms appear to be the result of an increased formation of acetaldehyde from alcohol* [18]." They also published a study of 83 patients in the period from December, 1947 to May, 1948 who were given disulfiram as a treatment for alcohol dependence. Since more than half the patients benefited, the drug was regarded as effective and promising. The treatment with disulfiram was thought to be an add-on to the general treatment of alcohol dependence [19].

Erik Glud, a young Danish physician at the New Haven (CT) Hospital in 1949 wrote a paper on Disulfiram use in American patients. As he pointed out, American drinking patterns were different from those in Scandinavian countries. At the annual meeting of the American Psychiatric Association in Montreal in May, 1949, a paper on disulfiram therapy by three physicians from Albany (NY) Hospital described the usefulness of the drug in the treatment of 21 patients, all habitual drinkers, over a period of 2–4 months. As a result of the treatment, 14 of the patients discontinued the use of alcohol entirely [20]. It was important they emphasized that the chief value of disulfiram laid in the fact that it paved the way for psychotherapeutic treatment. Disulfiram in conjunction with psychotherapy may prove superior to other methods of treatment of chronic alcohol dependence [21].

1.6 Early Disulfiram and Ethanol Metabolism Research

Investigation into the metabolism of alcohol and the effect of disulfiram in humans was a major research topic between 1945 and 1955. Many scientists focused on the clinical aspects, and others studied the biochemical and pharmacological aspects of disulfiram. Raby, a medical researcher, studied the disulfiram–ethanol reaction from a clinical point of view; and Erling Asmussen, a sports physiologist, did research on the pharmacological action of the acetaldehyde accumulated by the usage of disulfiram [22]. Jacobsen extensively studied the metabolism of ethanol, a topic of scientific importance at the time. The first extensive review on disufiram and ethanol metabolism was published in 1952. Ethanol metabolism had been studied by researchers as early as the 1920s and 1930s. Erik Widmark, a Swedish chemist, had established that the metabolism of practically all the ethanol ingested takes place in the liver, and that the enzymatic oxidation to acetic acid occurs with acetaldehyde as an intermediate product. However, little was known of the reaction mechanism with disulfiram [23]. According to the research at Copenhagen, ethanol was oxidized to acetaldehyde by means of the enzyme alcohol dehydrogenase (ADH) and the acetaldehyde is subsequently transformed into acetic acid by the action of another enzyme, aldehyde dehydrogenase (ALDH). The principal action of disulfiram was to block the action of ALDH, which results in an accumulation of acetaldehyde in the body [24] (Fig. 1.2).

The first researcher to establish the mechanism of action of Disulfiram as an ALDH inhibitor was Niels Ole Kjeldgaard, a 23-year graduate who went on to become a professor of molecular biology. In his research in 1949, he demonstrated that even in concentrations as small as 0.1 μg/ml disulfiram exerted a strong inhibition on the ALDH enzyme in the liver [25]. This contradicted the findings of Jacobsen and his team, which concluded that a much larger dose of disulfiram was required to block the transformation of ethanol to acetaldehyde. Hald and his collaborator Valdemar Larsen, a pharmacologist, discovered other substances besides disulfiram that act as inhibitors for ALDH. It had been known for some time that cyanamide provoked disagreeable symptoms in combination with alcohol, a similar effect was established for tetraethylthiuram monosulfide tetramethyl disulfide, and a few other compounds similar to disulfiram [26]. The research at that time propagated research not only in the metabolism of ethanol but also other areas of a related

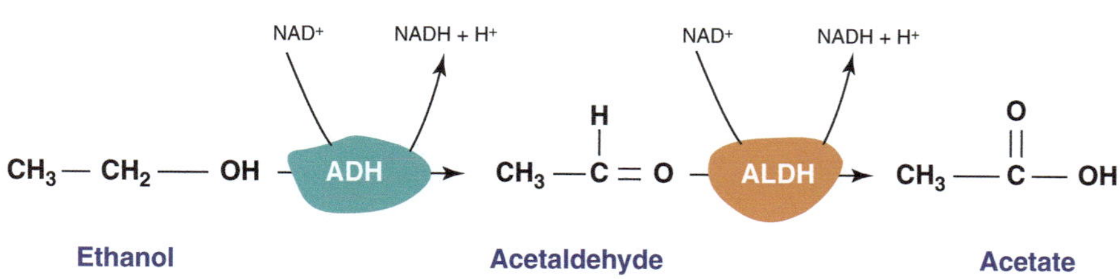

Fig. 1.2 Metabolic pathway of Ethanol and mechanism of action of Disulfiram. (Source—www.themedicalbiochemistrypage.org)

chemical, pharmacological and clinical nature. Around 150 papers on the subject were written between 1948 and 1953 and of these, about 40–50 were written by researchers from Denmark. The research also involved researchers from Sweden, the United States and Great Britain along with France, South Africa, and Canada [27]. Thus disulfiram was gaining international recognition.

1.7 Further Usage of Disulfiram in the Early Period

The treatment of alcohol dependence with disulfiram was introduced in the Scandinavian countries. In Denmark and Sweden, the drug was approved for medical prescriptions in early 1949. In spite of the reserved use by physicians, the public tended to see disulfiram as a wonder drug. Disulfiram was also the subject of many a newspaper headline at that time. By the 1950s, it had gained recognition as a permanent fixture in the treatment of alcohol misuse in the Danish circle. Disulfiram has always been considered a discovery of Denmark. In the beginning of the twenty-first century the total prescriptions per year in Denmark was five million daily doses, corresponding to an estimated 25,000 patients. In the United States, disulfiram (Antabuse) was approved by the Federal Drug Administration in 1951, followed by approval of newer drugs like naltextrone, 43 years later in 1994 and acamprosate in 2004. Disulfiram is underused in the United States with only 250,000 prescriptions per year. Disulfiram is still of major use in Denmark and the Scandinavian countries [28].

1.8 Discovery of the Non-Alcohol Uses of Disulfiram

The research in therapeutic properties of disulfiram other than those related to preventing excessive drinking found that it had a beneficial effect on symptoms caused by vitamin E deficiency [29]. A Danish odontologist, Jens Pindborg while working as a consultant, showed that certain dental diseases caused by lack of vitamin E could be cured by disulfiram [30]. Much research has recently been done on the therapeutic properties of the compound. It appears to have a potential in the treatment of human cancers and certain drug-resistant fungal infections [31, 32].

Thus the interesting history of the account of Disulfiram speaks about how the drug was discovered and gained the importance it has today in the management of alcohol dependence.

References

1. Suh JJ, Pettinati HM, Kampman KM, O'brien CP. The status of disulfiram: a half of a century later. J Clin Psychopharmacol. 2006;26(3):290–302.
2. Lundwall L, Baekeland F. Disulfiram treatment of alcoholism—a review. J Nerv Ment Dis. 1971;153(6):381–94.

3. Pal A, Pattanayak RD, Sagar R. Tracing the journey of disulfiram: from an unintended discovery to a treatment option for alcoholism. J Ment Health Hum Behav. 2015;20(1):41–3.
4. Ellis PM, Dronsfield AT. Antabuse's diamond anniversary: still sparkling on? Drug Alcohol Rev. 2013;32(4):342–4.
5. Billet SL. Antabuse therapy. Alcoholism: the total treatment approach. Springfield, IL: Charles C. Thomas; 1968.
6. Holmberg B, Sjöström B. Toxicological aspects of chemical hazards in the rubber industry. J Toxicol Environ Health. 1980;6(5–6):1201–9.
7. Tamai H, Yokoyama A, Okuyama K, Takahashi H, Maruyama K, Suzuki Y, Ishii H. Comparison of cyanamide and disulfiram in effects on liver function. Alcohol Clin Exp Res. 2000;24(4 Suppl):97S–9S.
8. Landegren J, Borglund E, Storgårds K. Treatment of scabies with disulfiram and benzyl benzoate emulsion: a controlled study. Acta Derm Venereol. 1978;59(3):274–6.
9. Jacobsen E. Deaths of alcoholic patients treated with disulfiram (tetraethylthiuram disulfide) in Denmark. Q J Stud Alcohol. 1952;13(1):16–26.
10. Hald J, Jacobsen E, Larsen V. Formation of acetaldehyde in the organism in relation to dosage of antabuse (tetraethylthiuram-disulphide) and to alcohol-concentration in blood. Basic Clin Pharmacol Toxicol. 1949;5(2):179–88.
11. Jacobsen E. The pharmacology of antabuse (tetraethylthiuramdisulphide). Addiction. 1950;47(1):26–40.
12. Jacobsen E, Larsen V. Site of the formation of acetaldehyde after ingestion of antabuse (tetraethylthiuramdisulphide) and alcohol. Basic Clin Pharmacol Toxicol. 1949;5(3):285–91.
13. Jacobsen E, Martensen-Larsen O. Treatment of alcoholism with tetraethylthiuram disulfide (Antabus®). JAMA. 1949;139(14):918–22.
14. Jacobsen E. Is acetaldehyde an intermediary product in normal metabolism? Biochim Biophys Acta. 1950;4:330–4.
15. Wright C, Moore RD. Disulfiram treatment of alcoholism. Am J Med. 1990;88(6):647–55.
16. Hald J, Jacobsen E, Larsen V. The sensitizing effect of tetraethylthiuramdisulphide (antabuse) to ethylalcohol. Basic Clin Pharmacol Toxicol. 1948;4(3–4):285–96.
17. Hald J, Jacobsen E. A drug sensitising the organism to ethyl alcohol. Lancet. 1948;252(6539):1001–4.
18. Hald J, Jacobsen E, Larsen V. The antabuse effect of some compound. Related to antabuse and cyanamide. Basic Clin Pharmacol Toxicol. 1952;8(4):329–37.
19. Petersen EN. The pharmacology and toxicology of disulfiram and its metabolites. Acta Psychiatr Scand. 1992;86(S369):7–13.
20. Glud E. The treatment of alcoholic patients in Denmark with antabuse with suggestions for its trial in the United States. Q J Stud Alcohol. 1949;10(2):185–90.
21. Miller WR, Walters ST, Bennett ME. How effective is alcoholism treatment in the United States? J Stud Alcohol. 2001;62(2):211–20.
22. Asmussen E, Hald J, Jacobsen E, Jørgensen G. Studies on the effect of tetraethylthiuramdisulphide (antabuse) and alcohol on respiration and circulation in normal human subjects. Basic Clin Pharmacol Toxicol. 1948;4(3–4):297–304.
23. Jacobsen E. The metabolism of ethyl alcohol. Nature. 1952;169(4303):645–7.
24. Vallari RC, Pietruszko R. Human aldehyde dehydrogenase: mechanism of inhibition of disulfiram. Science. 1982;216(4546):637–9.
25. Kjeldgaard NO. Inhibition of aldehyde oxidase from liver by tetraethylthiuramdisulphide (antabuse). Basic Clin Pharmacol Toxicol. 1949;5(4):397–403.
26. Johansson B. A review of the pharmacokinetics and pharmacodynamics of disulfiram and its metabolites. Acta Psychiatr Scand. 1992;86(S369):15–26.
27. Kragh H. From disulfiram to antabuse: the invention of a drug. Bull Hist Chem. 2008;33(2):82–8.
28. Carroll KM, Nich C, Ball SA, McCance E, Rounsavile BJ. Treatment of cocaine and alcohol dependence with psychotherapy and disulfiram. Addiction. 1998;93(5):713–27.

29. Aaes-Jørgensen E, Dam H, Granados H. The influence of antabuse (tetraethylthiuramdisulphide) and methylene blue on certain vitamin E deficiency symptoms and on growth in rats. Basic Clin Pharmacol Toxicol. 1951;7(2):171–80.
30. Dogterom P, Mulder GJ, Nagelkerke JF. Lipid peroxidation-dependent and -independent protein thiol modifications in isolated rat hepatocytes: differential effects of vitamin E and disulfiram. Chem-Biol Interact. 1989;71(2–3):291–306.
31. Wang W, McLeod HL, Cassidy J. Disulfiram-mediated inhibition of NF-κB activity enhances cytotoxicity of 5-fluorouracil in human colorectal cancer cell lines. Int J Cancer. 2003;104(4):504–11.
32. Sauna ZE, Shukla S, Ambudkar SV. Disulfiram, an old drug with new potential therapeutic uses for human cancers and fungal infections. Mol Biosyst. 2005;1(2):127–34.

Disulfiram: Pharmacology and Mechanism of Action

2

2.1 Introduction

This chapter aims to provide a basic overview of the clinical pharmacology and mechanism of action of disulfiram as it has been understood over the past seven decades. The chapter is aimed at clinical utility rather than just pharmacological details, and all facets of the pharmacokinetics, pharmacodynamics and mechanism of action of disulfiram are covered. Drugs have been developed over the years for the long-term management of alcohol dependence and are used as adjuncts to behaviour therapies, psychotherapy and psychosocial interventions. Disulfiram belongs to a class of drugs called (acetaldehyde dehydrogenase) ALDH inhibitors and is used clinically as an alcohol-deterrent agent. These drugs are known to convert the effect of alcohol from a pleasant to an unpleasant one [1]. Among these drugs, calcium carbimide and disulfiram are the most effective. They produce an accumulation of acetaldehyde at levels that become uncomfortable even after ingestion of small amounts of alcohol and thereby force the person not to drink any alcohol at all, promoting a forced abstinence [2].

2.2 Mechanism of Action of Disulfiram

In 1948, Hald and Jacobsen described for the first time a probable mode of action of disulfiram, resulting from an increase in acetaldehyde levels in both plasma and breath on ingestion of alcohol after consumption of the drug. Acetaldehyde is primarily responsible for the effects, probably owing to its release of mediators, which is histamine. The blood of alcohol-dependent patients appears to be more susceptible to this releasing action and thus disulfiram helps in the inhibition of further drinking via the disulfiram–ethanol reaction [3]. The release of acetaldehyde produces flushing of the skin, owing to cutaneous vasodilatation and hypotension due to reduced diastolic blood pressure with reflex tachycardia, breathlessness, tachypnoea, feeling a warm sensation, palpitations, anxiety, panic, headache, nausea and

A. De Sousa, *Disulfiram*, https://doi.org/10.1007/978-981-32-9876-7_2

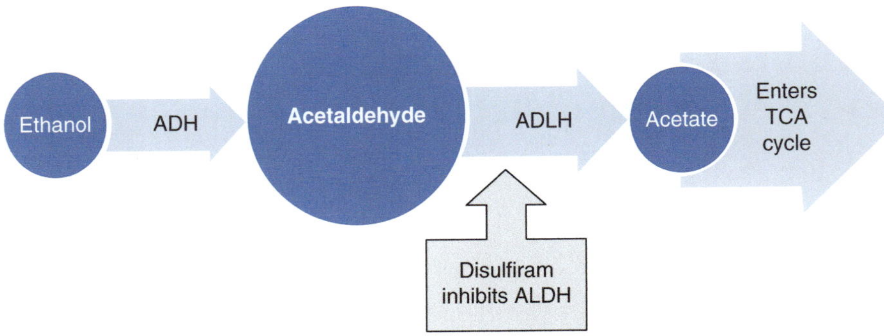

Fig. 2.1 Mechanism of action of Disulfiram. (Source—www.file.scirp.org—open access)

vomiting. The intensity and duration of this response is directly correlated to the time for which blood acetaldehyde concentrations are high. There is however a great inter-individual and intra-individual variation in the acetaldehyde-mediated reaction via disulfiram. Thus different individuals show different degrees of reaction, and the same individual may show a strong and intense reaction at one time and a milder response at another instance. These effects are also linked to variations in the form and isoenzymes of acetaldehyde dehydrogenase [4]. Studies have demonstrated that some Oriental populations lack isozyme ALDH-1, the low K_m isozyme, which is the crucial one for acetaldehyde metabolism. There are studies that show that the prevalence of ALDH-1 deficiency varies between 2% and 5% in Orientals compared to 30% and 40% in normal controls [5]. This may suggest that the impaired metabolism of acetaldehyde significantly reduces the risk of an alcohol problem developing. The principle on which disulfiram works, the unpleasant reaction contingent on alcohol ingestion above a certain low limit, appears to afford a degree of life-long protection against the development of alcoholism [6]. Studies have also reported that female subjects have lower levels of ALDH enzymes compared to males and hence may need lower doses of disulfiram to achieve control (Fig. 2.1) [7].

2.3 Disulfiram Metabolism in Human Subjects

It has been known for many years that disulfiram is extensively metabolized in the liver of alcohol-dependent subjects [8]. The main metabolite is diethyldithiomethylcarbamate (Me-DDC) which was first described in 1972 in animals [9] and in 1977 [10] in human subjects, respectively. This metabolite has similar alcohol-sensitizing properties as disulfiram in vivo [11]. Figure 2.2 describes the metabolic pathway of disulfiram in the human body and the intermediate compounds that are generated, most of which have similar properties to that of disulfiram. Of these diethylthiocarbamic acid methyl ester (Me-DTC) is the only

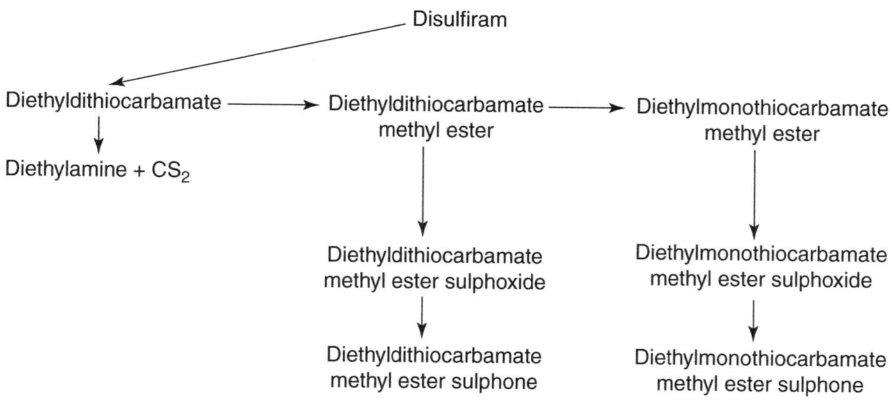

Fig. 2.2 The Metabolic Pathway of Disulfiram. (Source—free for use under https://creativecommons.org/licenses/by/4.0/)

metabolite that is rapid in its effect after alcohol ingestion and is easily detectable in plasma after disulfiram ingestion [12]. Concentrations of Me-DTC were 3–10 times higher than those of Me-DDC in studies [13]. Researchers have found that Me-DTC is active both parenterally and orally in animal studies [14]. It also actively inhibits ALDH in animal experiments. Rapid onset of action post Me-DTC injection than after disulfiram has been reported, though the biochemical differences between Me-DTC and disulfiram may be responsible for these variances [15]. Me-DTC has a much higher potency than either Me-DDC or disulfiram. The long-lasting effect of Me-DTC in studies has been attributed to irreversible enzyme inhibition [16].

2.4 Disulfiram and Its Action via Dopamine

High doses of disulfiram have been reported to inhibit cerebrospinal levels of enzyme dopamine β-hydroxylase in animal experiments [17]. The results with therapeutic doses in humans vary across various studies [18]. Patients with very low activity of dopamine β-hydroxylase appear to be sensitive to disulfiram and they may develop a transient psychotic condition probably because of an increased ratio between dopamine and noradrenaline in the brain [19]. This is also recognized now as one of the mechanisms for disulfiram reducing the effect of cocaine via dopamine and thus being used as a drug of choice for cocaine dependence [20]. The transient psychosis seen with disulfiram is reversible and clears off when the drug is withdrawn. It is also noteworthy to mention that more cases of psychosis with disulfiram have been reported in Asian subjects and very rarely in the west. Disulfiram seems to be a weak inhibitor of this enzyme again accounting for differences in its action across cocaine-dependent subjects (Fig. 2.3) [21].

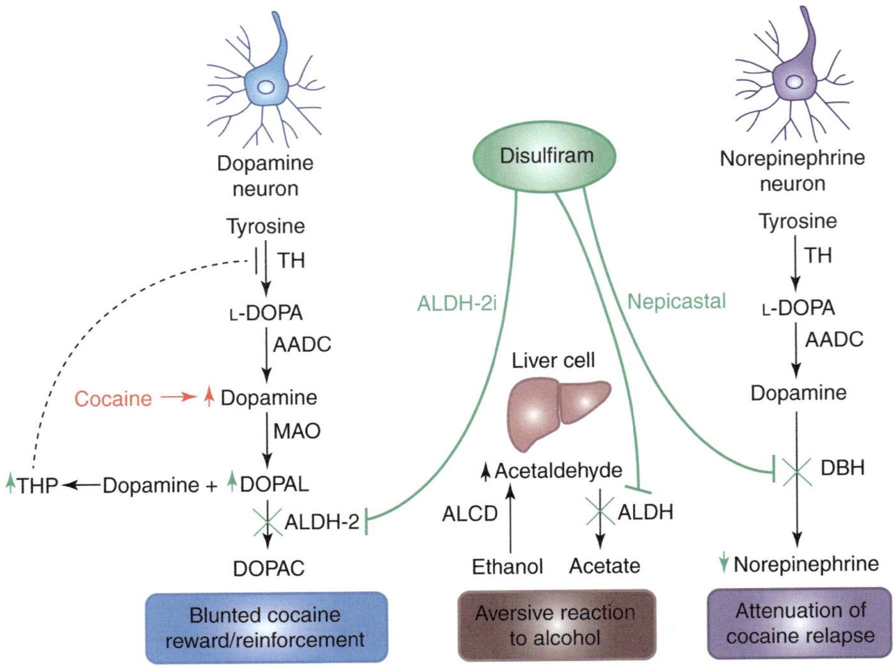

Fig. 2.3 Disulfiram effect on Dopamine metabolism. (Free for use from https://www.tumblr.com/tagged/antabuse)

2.5 Absorption and Biotransformation of Disulfiram

After oral ingestion, disulfiram is metabolized to diethyldithiocarbamic acid (DDC) in the strongly acidic juice of the stomach [22]. DDC is extremely unstable in acidic solutions and decomposes rapidly into carbon disulphide (CS,) and diethylamine (DEA) [8]. DDC forms a bis(diethy1dithiocarbamato) copper complex (Cu(DDC). Cu(DDC) is more acid-stable than is DDC, and unlike DDC is also neutral and extremely hydrophobic, which permits absorption along the entire length of the upper gastrointestinal tract. Accordingly, it could be claimed that systemic absorption is not restricted to the parent drug but also includes CU(DDC) [23]. Effervescent forms of DSF increase its bioavailability and show better results than normal disulfiram [24]. Enteric-coated tablets of disulfiram help the transport of intact DDC through the stomach and into the alkaline part of the small intestine. DDC is a highly polar and hydrophilic compound, and a hydrophobic complex with cupric ions must be formed for better action [25]. Disulfiram is rapidly absorbed from the human gastrointestinal tract and the amount excreted in faeces varies from 10% to 30%. Around 75–85% of the oral dose is absorbed [26].

After distribution across the gastrointestinal mucosa into blood, disulfiram is rapidly reduced to its monomer DDC, by the action of endogenous thiols and the glutathione reductase system [27]. Disulfiram is not easily detectable in blood at therapeutic doses, and the difficulties experienced in attempts to isolate, detect and quantify DSF in blood samples were caused by its dithiocarbamate structure, i.e. owing to its electrophilicity, it rapidly undergoes a redox disulphide interchange reaction with endogenous thiols [28]. It is now possible to measure and quantify blood concentration of intact disulfiram after a therapeutic dose. However, detectable levels have been noted only during the second week of treatment [29].

2.6 Distribution and Excretion of Disulfiram

After absorption, disulfiram and its metabolites are uniformly distributed throughout the body in various tissues. Disulfiram has been detected across blood, liver, kidney, heart, adrenal, thyroid, pancreas, testes, spleen, marrow and muscle using radioactive tagging [30]. The distribution in various organs varies, probably depending on which types of enzyme systems are involved and present in each tissue [31]. Disulfiram and DDC are bound with various proteins. Me-DTC is highly bound to albumin. The metabolites of disulfiram are mainly excreted via the kidney, feces and the lungs [32]. This is also the basis why breath analyzers and urine estimations have been used in assessing compliance with disulfiram therapy.

2.7 Aldehyde Dehydrogenase Enzymes

Acetaldehyde is the first major metabolite of ethanol oxidation. It has been suggested that the adverse effects of acetaldehyde results from lipid peroxidation, generation of highly reactive free radicals, inactivation of various enzymes and by irreversible binding to proteins and other cells constituents, with impairment of cell membrane functions as a consequence [33]. Instantaneous metabolism is possible by further oxidation of acetaldehyde to form acetate which is catalyzed by ALDH [34]. There are four different isozyme forms of ALDH that have been described in humans. They show varied distribution, and two of them (ALDH 1 and ALDH 2) are mainly found in the liver [35]. They are the main enzymes for the metabolic oxidation of acetaldehyde. Inhibition of ALDH 1 by disulfiram and its metabolites brings about a dramatic rise in the blood concentration of acetaldehyde in humans, and this is considered to be the rationale for most, but not all, of the distressing physical symptoms of the Disulfiram–Ethanol Reaction (DER), i.e. hypotension, tachycardia, nausea, dyspnoea and flushing [36]. Disulfiram only partially inactivates ALDH 1 in vitro, whereas the activity of ALDH 2 is almost completely lost. It is suggested that ALDH 2 does not become implicated in the oxidation of acetaldehyde until ALDH 1 is sufficiently inactivated, thus promoting an increase in the blood concentration of acetaldehyde upon the ingestion of ethanol [37]. Moreover, a close relationship was found between the dose, the DER, high blood concentrations of acetaldehyde and measurable concentrations of Me-DDC [38]. It is also possible that different metabolites of DSF inactivate different isozymes of ALDH [39].

2.8 Pharmacokinetics of Disulfiram

Basic pharmacokinetic studies have been carried out with disulfiram. Researchers have noted a marked inter-subject variation in the plasma concentrations of disulfiram and its metabolites [40]. The biochemical effects of a daily increased dose of disulfiram (100, 200 and 300 mg), followed by ethanol provocation of a DER, were investigated in human volunteers. The drug was not detectable in any of the blood samples. However, the 100 mg dose produced detectable plasma concentrations of Me-DDC in all the subjects. In addition, plasma concentrations peaked in all groups at the optimal dose. A relation between elevated Me-DDC plasma concentrations and increased formation of blood acetaldehyde was also noted. The mean plasma concentrations of Me-DTC at the steady state were proportional to the DSF doses given, when compared within groups at the different dose levels [41]. These results suggest that the plasma concentration of Me-DTC may serve as a marker not only of the oxidative metabolic capacity of the liver but also of the therapeutic effectiveness of disulfiram treatment in patients. In low oxidizing patients a 100 mg dose may be sufficient, but in a high oxidizing patient we may need a 300–500 mg dose [42].

In patients with normal liver function and receiving clinical disulfiram treatment, erythrocyte ALDH is inactivated within a period of 3–5 days and the Me-DTC plasma concentrations are consistent with those of healthy volunteers. In patients with alcoholic liver disease and receiving disulfiram 200–400 mg per day, the inactivation of ALDH may be hampered by the limited oxidizing capacity of the cytochromes [43]. This might lead to drug therapeutic tolerance. A study on alcoholic and non-alcoholic liver disease subjects has shown significant decline in ALDH-1 activity in alcoholic patients. Acetaldehyde detoxification changes from ALDH-1 to the ALDH-2 oxidation pathway, thus causing intracellular accumulation of acetaldehyde which may further contribute to liver cell damage. Hence, patients tolerant to disulfiram may have impaired microsomal cytochrome P450 metabolizing capacity depending on elevated acetaldehyde and may produce less Me-DTC causing a weak disulfiram–ethanol reaction response [44].

2.9 Measuring Compliance When on Disulfiram Therapy

Pharmacological compliance is a must along with supervised medication to ensure success of a disulfiram treatment programme. It becomes very difficult for clinicians to ascertain compliance when medication is unsupervised. This is a very important aspect of the treatment programme as many patients with alcohol dependence relapse due to non-compliance on disulfiram [45]. Thus there has been an interest in the development of compliance tests based either on chemical measurements of metabolites or on measurements of the pharmacodynamic effect. Carbon disulphide in the breath can be detected for less than 24 h [46] and diethylamine in the urine for about the same time [47]. Among the metabolites of disulfiram, only Me-DTC appears reasonable to use for quantitative purposes and in this case the blood sample should be taken at the time the plasma concentration reaches its maximum i.e. 4–8 h after dosing [47]. Carbon disulfide blood levels may be estimated using gas chromatography, but it is a pain staking procedure when the number of subjects are more.

Theoretically an indirect way to assess the extent of ALDH-1 activity could be cutaneous vasodilatation in the ethanol patch test. A positive outcome in this test correlated closely to the lack of ALDH-1 isoenzyme. As disulfiram inhibits this enzyme, such an inhibition may also be supposed to be found in the skin as well [48]. Direct measurement of the liver mitochondria ALDH obtained by biopsy is the most relevant test to perform, but is for obvious reasons inadvisable [49].

Ethylglucuronide (EtG), a direct alcohol metabolite, has been reported to be a useful urinary marker of recent alcohol consumption. After consumption of even small amounts of alcohol, EtG becomes positive, and alcohol consumption could be detected up to 80 h after the elimination of alcohol from the body. However, detection time for EtG also depends on the dose of alcohol consumed. Thus, EtG has been shown to detect alcohol consumption with high sensitivity and specificity. Small-scale studies have proposed the role of EtG levels in urine as a marker of alcohol abstinence when on disulfiram treatment [50, 51].

Breath tests using breath analyzer equipment are being designed to assess compliance when on disulfiram therapy. The analyzer that has been studied is a hand-held breath analyzer, the Zenalyser™ (Zenics Medical), to identify alcohol-dependent patients receiving disulfiram therapy. The breath samples are analyzed for the combined concentration of carbon disulphide and acetone produced from the metabolism of disulfiram. It is very specific and sensitive. However, it is worth mentioning that breath levels fade if the patient is irregular, and patients on a daily disulfiram treatment regimen shall do better on breath analysis compared to those on a thrice weekly regimen [52].

The Zenalyser® has been used in the following way i.e. a patient blows into the instrument, connects it to a computer and the result is exported to the treating team, a process that takes <45 s from start to finish. The treating team reads the result and emails the patient back, which takes no more than a couple of minutes depending on the content of the email. Alternatively, the Zenalyser can be kept at the treating base, and patients can attend at frequent intervals to provide breath samples. Feedback from families and patients shows that they appreciate this technique, being reassured that when a patient leaves the safety of a detoxification or rehabilitation unit the clinical team continues with daily contact. Family members too, with permission, can read the emails from the treating team and be reassured that disulfiram has been taken and that the levels are in the therapeutic range. This is a very useful apparatus in over-worked and under-resourced centres where compliance may be monitored using a breath test but long-term clinical studies with the technique are still awaited [53].

2.10 Drug Interactions with Disulfiram

A large variety of drugs like cephalosporin antibiotics [54], amitriptyline [55], chloral hydrate [56], sulphonylurea hypoglycemic agents [57], metronidazole [58] and calcium carbimide [59] have been reported to produce DER-like reactions in combination with alcohol. Most of those drugs exert their action by inhibiting ALDH activity, but generally to a lesser degree, with a resulting DER that is milder than one which occurs with disulfiram [60]. A more serious problem arises with drugs that are administered in combination or connection with disulfiram therapy. The dose of disulfiram may have to be reduced when these drugs are administered concomitantly by physicians who are unaware of the combined effect on ALDH.

Disulfiram in human subjects is known via the cytochrome p450 system to raise phenytoin levels when both are administered together and phenytoin toxicity has been reported in subjects when the two drugs are used together [61]. Barbiturates and a numerous benzodiazepines e.g. chlordiazepoxide and diazepam, which are mainly metabolized by oxidation, are susceptible to reduced clearance, whereas others, like lorazepam and oxazepam which are excreted as glucuronides, are unaffected [62]. It has also been shown that disulfiram prolongs the metabolism of caffeine and thus coffee drinkers may be more alert than non-coffee drinkers when on disulfiram therapy [63]. Theophylline and the aminophylline bronchodilators are subjected to dose-related inhibitory metabolism by the action of disulfiram. Inhibition of its oxidative metabolism results in decreased plasma clearance and dose reduction by 50% is therefore recommended to prevent toxicity [64].

There are some reports of onset of disulfiram-like reactions related to topical administration. When combined with ethanol, tacrolimus and pimecrolimus, cream and ointment, respectively, may cause erythematosus flushing even after consuming a small amount of beer or wine [65]. Disulfiram-like reactions have been reported in patients who consume alcoholic beverages while being treated with furazolidone [66]. The antiandrogen nilutamide has been associated with alcohol intolerance that takes the form of a slight disulfiram-like reaction, with hot flashes and skin rash being the main symptoms [67]. When medications that produce disulfiram-like reactions are prescribed or dispensed, patients should be instructed to avoid medicines and other products containing alcohol, such as cough syrups, fermented vinegar, sauces and lotions. Medicinal products containing ethanol, as elixirs, have been implicated in some cases of acetaldehyde syndrome [68].

2.11 Conclusion

This chapter thus has provided an overview of the basic clinical pharmacology and mechanism of action of disulfiram. The chapter has looked at human subjects much more than animal experiments and has focused on the clinical utility of the pharmacology of disulfiram. Various aspects of disulfiram metabolism, absorption, clearance and methods to improve disulfiram compliance have been discussed along with the propensity of many over-the-counter medications to cause a disulfiram-like reaction when administered with alcohol.

References

1. Petersen EN. The pharmacology and toxicology of disulfiram and its metabolites. Acta Psychiatr Scand. 1992;86(S369):7–13.
2. Peachey JE, Brien JF, Roach CA, Loomis CW. A comparative review of the pharmacological and toxicological properties of disulfiram and calcium carbimide. J Clin Psychopharmacol. 1981;1(1):21–6.

3. Kitson TM. The disulfiram—ethanol reaction: a review. J Stud Alcohol. 1977;38(1):96–113.
4. Savas MC, Güllü İH. Disulfiram–ethanol test reaction: significance of supervision. Ann Pharmacother. 1997;31(3):374–5.
5. Harada S, Agarwal DP, Goedde HW. Mechanism of alcohol sensitivity and disulfiram-ethanol reaction. Subst Alcohol Actions Misuse. 1982;3(1–2):107–15.
6. Fuller RK, Branchey L, Brightwell DR, Derman RM, Emrick CD, Iber FL, James KE, Lacoursiere RB, Lee KK, Lowenstam I, Maany I. Disulfiram treatment of alcoholism: a veterans administration cooperative study. JAMA. 1986;256(11):1449–55.
7. Nich C, McCance-Katz EF, Petrakis IL, Cubells JF, Rounsaville BJ, Carroll KM. Sex differences in cocaine-dependent individuals' response to disulfiram treatment. Addict Behav. 2004;29(6):1123–8.
8. Yourick JJ, Faiman MD. Comparative aspects of disulfiram and its metabolites in the disulfiram-ethanol reaction in the rat. Biochem Pharmacol. 1989;38(3):413–21.
9. Johansson B, Stankiewicz Z. Inhibition of erythrocyte aldehyde dehydrogenase activity and elimination kinetics of diethyldithiocarbamic acid methyl ester and its monothio analogue after administration of single and repeated doses of disulfiram to man. Eur J Clin Pharmacol. 1989;37(2):133–8.
10. Cobby J, Mayersohn M, Selliah S. Methyl diethyldithiocarbamate, a metabolite of disulfiram in man. Life Sci. 1977;21(7):937–41.
11. Petersen EN. Pharmacological effects of diethylthiocarbamic acid methyl ester, the active metabolite of disulfiram? Eur J Pharmacol. 1989;166(3):419–25.
12. Rahman MA, Grunberg NE, Mueller GP. Disulfiram causes sustained behavioral and biochemical effects in rats. Pharmacol Biochem Behav. 1997;56(3):409–15.
13. Johansson B. Distribution of disulfiram and its chief metabolites over erythrocyte cell membranes and inactivation of erythrocyte aldehyde dehydrogenase activity. Basic Clin Pharmacol Toxicol. 1990;66(2):104–8.
14. Petersen EN, Johansson B. Characterization of a third step active metabolite off disulfiram, diethylthiocarbamic acid methyl ester. Eur J Pharmacol. 1990;183(2):563–4.
15. Johansson B, Angelo HR, Christensen JK, Møller IW, Rønsted P. Dose-effect relationship of disulfiram in human volunteers. II: A study of the relation between the disulfiram-alcohol reaction and plasma concentrations of acetaldehyde, diethyldithiocarbamic acid methyl ester, and erythrocyte aldehyde dehydrogenase activity. Basic Clin Pharmacol Toxicol. 1991;68(3):166–70.
16. Strömme JH. Metabolism of disulfiram and diethyldithiocarbamate in rats with demonstration of an in vivo ethanol-induced inhibition of the glucuronic acid conjugation of the thiol. Biochem Pharmacol. 1965;14(4):393–410.
17. Ewing JA, Rouse BA, Mueller RA, Silver D. Can dopamine beta-hydroxylase levels predict adverse reactions to disulfiram? Alcohol Clin Exp Res. 1978;2(1):93–4.
18. Schroeder JP, Cooper DA, Schank JR, Lyle MA, Gaval-Cruz M, Ogbonmwan YE, Pozdeyev N, Freeman KG, Iuvone PM, Edwards GL, Holmes PV. Disulfiram attenuates drug-primed reinstatement of cocaine seeking via inhibition of dopamine β-hydroxylase. Neuropsychopharmacology. 2010;35(12):2440–8.
19. Ewing JA, Mueller RA, Rouse BA, Silver D. Low levels of dopamine beta-hydroxylase and psychosis. Am J Psychiatry. 1977;134(8):927–33.
20. Kosten TR, Wu G, Huang W, Harding MJ, Hamon SC, Lappalainen J, Nielsen DA. Pharmacogenetic randomized trial for cocaine abuse: disulfiram and dopamine β-hydroxylase. Biol Psychiatry. 2013;73(3):219–24.
21. Gaval-Cruz M, Schroeder JP, Liles LC, Javors MA, Weinshenker D. Effects of disulfiram and dopamine beta-hydroxylase knockout on cocaine-induced seizures. Pharmacol Biochem Behav. 2008;89(4):556–62.
22. Yourick JJ, Faiman MD. Disulfiram metabolism as a requirement for the inhibition of rat liver mitochondrial low Km aldehyde dehydrogenase. Biochem Pharmacol. 1991;42(7):1361–6.
23. Johansson B, Stankiewicz Z. Bis-(diethyldithiocarbamato) copper complex: a new metabolite of disulfiram? Biochem Pharmacol. 1985;34(16):2989–91.
24. Andersen MP. Lack of bioequivalence between disulfiram formulations. Acta Psychiatr Scand. 1992;86(S369):31–5.

25. Eneanya DI, Bianchine JR, Duran DO, Andresen BD. The actions and metabolic fate of disulfiram. Annu Rev Pharmacol Toxicol. 1981;21(1):575–96.
26. Cobby J, Mayersohn M, Selliah S. Disposition kinetics in dogs of diethyldithiocarbamate, a metabolite of disulfiram. J Pharmacokinet Biopharm. 1978;6(5):369–87.
27. Brien JF, Loomis CW. Disposition and pharmacokinetics of disulfiram and calcium carbimide (calcium cyanamide). Drug Metab Rev. 1983;14(1):113–26.
28. MacKerell AD, Vallari RC, Pietruszko R. Human mitochondrial aldehyde dehydrogenase inhibition by diethyldithiocarbamic acid methanethiol mixed disulfide: a derivative of disulfiram. FEBS Lett. 1985;179(1):77–81.
29. Brewer C. How effective is the standard dose of disulfiram? A review of the alcohol-disulfiram reaction in practice. Br J Psychiatry. 1984;144(2):200–2.
30. Faiman MD, Artman L, Haya K. Disulfiram distribution and elimination in the rat after oral and intraperitoneal administration. Alcohol Clin Exp Res. 1980;4(4):412–9.
31. Hart BW, Yourick JJ, Faiman MD. S-methyl-N,N-diethylthiolcarbamate: a disulfiram metabolite and potent rat liver mitochondrial low K m aldehyde dehydrogenase inhibitor. Alcohol. 1990;7(2):165–9.
32. Yourick JJ, Faiman MD. Diethyldithiocarbamic acid-methyl ester: a metabolite of disulfiram and its alcohol sensitizing properties in the disulfiram-ethanol reaction. Alcohol. 1987;4(6):463–7.
33. Crabb DW, Edenberg HJ, Bosron WF, Li TK. Genotypes for aldehyde dehydrogenase deficiency and alcohol sensitivity. The inactive ALDH2 (2) allele is dominant. J Clin Investig. 1989;83(1):314–20.
34. Bosron WF, Li TK. Genetic polymorphism of human liver alcohol and aldehyde dehydrogenases, and their relationship to alcohol metabolism and alcoholism. Hepatology. 1986;6(3):502–10.
35. Harada S, Misawa SH, Agarwal DP, Goedde HW. Liver alcohol dehydrogenase and aldehyde dehydrogenase in the Japanese: isozyme variation and its possible role in alcohol intoxication. Am J Hum Genet. 1980;32(1):8–17.
36. Goedde HW, Agarwal DP, Eckey R, Harada S. Population genetic and family studies on aldehyde dehydrogenase deficiency and alcohol sensitivity. Alcohol. 1985;2(3):383–90.
37. Harada S, Agarwal DP, Goedde HW. Aldehyde dehydrogenase deficiency as cause of facial flushing reaction to alcohol in Japanese. Lancet. 1981;318(8253):982.
38. Veverka KA, Johnson KL, Mays DC, Lipsky JJ, Naylor S. Inhibition of aldehyde dehydrogenase by disulfiram and its metabolite methyl diethylthiocarbamoyl-sulfoxide. Biochem Pharmacol. 1997;53(4):511–8.
39. Rex DK, Bosron WF, Smialek JE, Li TK. Alcohol and aldehyde dehydrogenase isoenzymes in North American Indians. Alcohol Clin Exp Res. 1985;9(2):147–52.
40. Fuller RK, Gordis E. Does disulfiram have a role in alcoholism treatment today? Addiction. 2004;99(1):21–4.
41. Johansson B, Angelo HR, Christensen JK, Mdller IW, Rdnsted P. Dose-effect relationship of disulfiram in human volunteers: a study of the relation between the disulfiram-alcohol reaction and plasma concentrations of acetaldehyde, diethyldithiocarbamic acid methyl ester, and erythrocyte aldehyde dehydrogenase activity. Pharmacol Toxicol. 1991;68:166–70.
42. Mays DC, Nelson AN, Lam-Holt J, Fauq AH, Lipsky JJ. S-methyl-N,N-diethylthiocarbamate sulfoxide and S-methyl-N,N-diethylthiocarbamate sulfone, two candidates for the active metabolite of disulfiram. Alcohol Clin Exp Res. 1996;20(3):595–600.
43. Brady JF, Xiao F, Wang MH, Li Y, Ning SM, Gapac JM, Yang CS. Effects of disulfiram on hepatic P450IIE1, other microsomal enzymes, and hepatotoxicity in rats. Toxicol Appl Pharmacol. 1991;108(2):366–73.
44. Lipsky JJ, Shen ML, Naylor S. In vivo inhibition of aldehyde dehydrogenase by disulfiram. Chem Biol Interact. 2001;130:93–102.
45. Allen JP, Litten RZ. Techniques to enhance compliance with disulfiram. Alcohol Clin Exp Res. 1992;16(6):1035–41.

46. Wells J, Koves E. Detection of carbon disulphide (a disulfiram metabolite) in expired air by gas chromatography. J Chromatogr. 1974;92(2):442–4.
47. Zaldívar-Machorro VJ, López-Ortiz M, Demare P, Regla I, Muñoz-Clares RA. The disulfiram metabolites S-methyl-N,N-diethyldithiocarbamoyl sulfoxide and S-methyl-N,N-diethylthiocarbamoyl sulfone irreversibly inactivate betaine aldehyde dehydrogenase from Pseudomonas aeruginosa, both in vitro and in situ, and arrest bacterial growth. Biochimie. 2011;93(2):286–95.
48. Murarnatsu T, Higuchi S, Shigernori K, Saito M, Sasao M, Harada S, Shigeta Y, Yamada K, Muraoka H, Takagi S, Maruyarna K. Ethanol patch test—a simple and sensitive method for identifying ALDH phenotype. Alcohol Clin Exp Res. 1989;13(2):229–31.
49. Ricciardi BR, Saunders JB, Williams R, Hopkinson DA. Identification of alcohol dehydrogenase and aldehyde dehydrogenase isoenzymes in human liver biopsy specimens. Clin Chem Acta. 1983;130(1):85–94.
50. Wurst FM, Wiesbeck GA, Metzger JW, Weinmann W, Graf M. On sensitivity, specificity, and the influence of various parameters on ethyl glucuronide levels in urine—results from the WHO/ISBRA study. Alcohol Clin Exp Res. 2004;28(8):1220–8.
51. Mutschler J, Grosshans M, Koopmann A, Mann K, Kiefer F, Hermann D. Urinary ethylglucuronide assessment in patients treated with disulfiram: a tool to improve verification of abstention and safety. Clin Neuropharmacol. 2010;33(6):285–7.
52. Fletcher K, Stone E, Mohamad MW, Faulder GC, Faulder RM, Jones K, Morgan D, Wegerdt J, Kelly M, Chick J. A breath test to assess compliance with disulfiram. Addiction. 2006;101(12):1705–10.
53. Fletcher K. Disulfiram and the Zenalyser®: teaching an old dog new tricks. Alcohol Alcohol. 2015;50(2):255–6.
54. Uri JV, Parks DB. Disulfiram-like reaction to certain cephalosporins. Ther Drug Monit. 1983;5(2):219–24.
55. Weathermon R, Crabb DW. Alcohol and medication interactions. Alcohol Res Health. 1999;23(1):40–54.
56. Chen Z, Zhang J, Stamler JS. Identification of the enzymatic mechanism of nitroglycerin bioactivation. Proc Natl Acad Sci U S A. 2002;99(12):8306–11.
57. Towell J, Garthwaite T, Wang R. Erythrocyte aldehyde dehydrogenase and disulfiram-like side effects of hypoglycemics and antianginals. Alcohol Clin Exp Res. 1985;9(5):438–42.
58. Visapää JP, Tillonen JS, Kaihovaara PS, Salaspuro MP. Lack of disulfiram-like reaction with metronidazole and ethanol. Ann Pharmacother. 2002;36(6):971–4.
59. Glatt MM. Disulfiram and citrated calcium carbimide in the treatment of alcoholism. Br J Psychiatry. 1959;105(439):476–81.
60. Karamanakos PN, Pappas P, Boumba VA, Thomas C, Malamas M, Vougiouklakis T, Marselos M. Pharmaceutical agents known to produce disulfiram-like reaction: effects on hepatic ethanol metabolism and brain monoamines. Int J Toxicol. 2007;26(5):423–32.
61. MacLeod SM, Sellers EM, Giles HG, Billings BJ, Martin PR, Greenblatt DJ, Marshman JA. Interaction of disulfiram with benzodiazepines. Clin Pharmacol Ther. 1978;24(5):583–9.
62. Abernethy DR, Greenblatt DJ, Ochs HR, Shader RI. Benzodiazepine drug-drug interactions commonly occurring in clinical practice. Curr Med Res Opin. 1984;8(Suppl 4):80–93.
63. Beach CA, Mays DC, Guiler RC, Jacober CH, Gerber N. Inhibition of elimination of caffeine by disulfiram in normal subjects and recovering alcoholics. Clin Pharmacol Ther. 1986;39(3):265–70.
64. Loi CM, Day JD, Jue SG, Bush ED, Costello P, Dewey LV, Vestal RE. Dose-dependent inhibition of theophylline metabolism by disulfiram in recovering alcoholics. Clin Pharmacol Ther. 1989;45(5):476–86.
65. Wilkin JK. Flushing reactions: consequences and mechanisms. Ann Intern Med. 1981;95(4):468–76.

66. Vasiliou V, Malamas M, Marselos M. The mechanism of alcohol intolerance produced by various therapeutic agents. Basic Clin Pharmacol Toxicol. 1986;58(5):305–10.
67. Singer EA, Golijanin DJ, Miyamoto H, Messing EM. Androgen deprivation therapy for prostate cancer. Expert Opin Pharmacother. 2008;9(2):211–28.
68. Kwentus J, Major LF. Disulfiram in the treatment of alcoholism; a review. J Stud Alcohol. 1979;40(5):428–46.

3 Disulfiram in the Management of Alcohol Dependence

3.1 Introduction

Disulfiram is an alcohol-deterrent agent used in the long-term management of alcohol dependence. Ethanol undergoes metabolism in the liver initially by alcohol dehydrogenase (ADH) forming acetaldehyde; this is removed from the body primarily by oxidation into acetate by acetaldehyde dehydrogenase (ALDH) [1] (Fig. 3.1), which finally enters the citric acid cycle. Disulfiram acts by inhibiting the enzyme ALDH via its metabolite *S*-methyl-*N*,*N*-diethyl-dithiocarbamate-sulphoxide [2], leading to accumulation of acetaldehyde in blood. This gives rise to various manifestations of disulfiram–ethanol reaction (DER) [3]. Since the inhibition of ALDH by disulfiram is irreversible, the DER will get terminated only after production of new ALDH once disulfiram is stopped. The new ALDH takes about a week's time to be produced. Hence patients should be advised to take alcohol only after 2 weeks of stopping disulfiram [4].

In addition to this, disulfiram also acts on the dopaminergic system, both disulfiram and its metabolite carbon disulfide leading to inhibition of dopamine

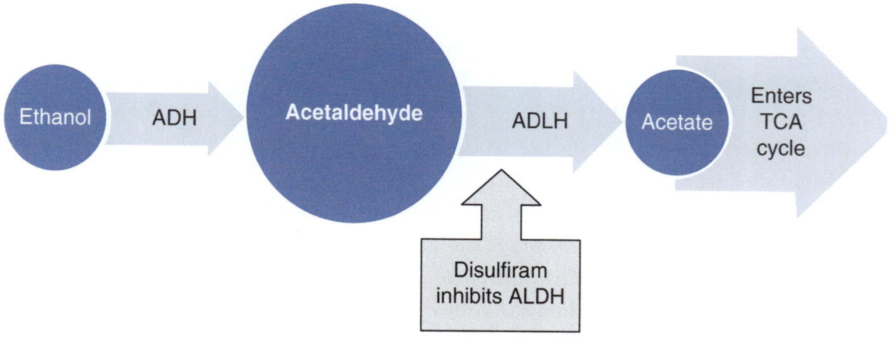

Fig. 3.1 Mechanism of action of disulfiram. (Source—Open access under www.file.scirp.org)

A. De Sousa, *Disulfiram*, https://doi.org/10.1007/978-981-32-9876-7_3

beta-hydroxylase (DBH) that leads to increase in the levels of dopamine [5]. Besides this action, disulfiram is also known to inhibit dopamine beta-hydroxylase leading to an increase in dopamine concentrations but decreased norepinephrine in the brain suggesting an anti-craving role of disulfiram in alcohol dependence [6, 7].

The present chapter is an overview of various studies of disulfiram in the management of alcohol dependence and provides the clinically relevant conclusions of these studies.

3.2 Studies of Disulfiram in Patients with Alcohol Dependence

The present section reviews some of the most important studies done on disulfiram in alcohol dependence. Disulfiram studies that involve combination with other pharmacological agents and in specific special populations like multiple substance abusers, adolescents and alcohol dependents with psychiatric comorbidity are reviewed in another chapter dedicated to the role of disulfiram in special populations.

In a recent meta-analysis of 11 randomized controlled trials with a total of 1527 patients, the researchers concluded that supervised disulfiram did have some effect on the short-term abstinence, days until relapse and number of drinking days when compared to placebo, no treatment or other treatments available for patients with alcohol dependence or abuse [8]. In another recent meta-analysis, that included 22 studies, the authors concluded that when comparing blind and open-label trials of disulfiram, only open-label trials showed a significant superiority over controls. Trials with blind designs showed no efficacy of disulfiram compared to controls and the drug was also more effective than the control condition when compared to naltrexone, acamprosate and to the no-disulfiram groups. The limitation of the study was 89% male subjects and huge heterogeneity of studies [9].

In a study that analyzed the effect of supervised disulfiram along with cognitive behaviour therapy (CBT) in 39 patients of alcohol dependence but reported only 20% and 26% rate of abstinence in the control and disulfiram group respectively. They concluded that supervised disulfiram therapy did not have any major impact on the treatment outcome in this disorder [10]. In one of the most cited disulfiram trials to date, the Veterans Affairs multisite cooperative study also showed that disulfiram and placebo-treated patients had similar outcomes. This study is the most quoted for disulfiram and its efficacy and itself mentions the need for supervised disulfiram therapy with the failure to include supervision of disulfiram therapy in his study as a serious limitation [11].

Medication non-adherence is often cited as a strong factor that impedes the effectiveness of disulfiram since many patients with alcohol dependence themselves stop the drug due to its impeding ability on drinking [12]. In a study on 210 patients of alcohol dependence who had voluntarily discontinued disulfiram treatment, it was found that none of these patients reported adverse events as a reason for discontinuing disulfiram treatment. Around 70% of their patients gave reasons such as 'a wish to drink again' or 'no need for treatment anymore'. It is likely that many patients often over-estimate their self-capacity to control substance intake and in this belief, stop disulfiram but also restart alcohol [13]. In other studies, only a small percentage (5–18%) of 345 alcohol-dependent inpatients discontinued disulfiram owing to side effects. Thus, it is not the side effects that lead to discontinuation of disulfiram, but the basic characteristics of alcohol dependence that lead to relapse [14].

It has been repeatedly emphasized that medication adherence and compliance with disulfiram can be increased easily with good psychoeducation, family support and supervised disulfiram therapy when administered by a family member [15]. Research suggests that the mode of action of disulfiram is a combined psychological deterrent action and a physiological deterrent action [16]. However, experiencing the disulfiram ethanol recation is not necessary for disulfiram's action and does not lead to better treatment outcome in effect [17].

In a long follow-up study (9 years from 1993–2002), authors studied the abstinence, relapse and lapse rates in patients with alcohol dependence during an outpatient long-term intensive therapy for alcoholics. This study was called the OLITA trial and is one of the few studies where sham disulfiram therapy was compared to actual disulfiram therapy. An abstinence rate of more than 50% was noted across both groups despite the long duration of the study. This indicates the role of long-term deterrent (disulfiram) therapy in the management of alcohol dependence along with a psychological component that plays a role in the mechanism of disulfiram's action. This is because an assumption of just being on disulfiram therapy in the sham group led to similar abstinence rates compared to actual disulfiram therapy [18]. The same set of researchers also published a review paper that emphasizes the role of disulfiram as an adjunct to psychotherapy in alcoholism treatment [19]. Another article has reviewed disulfiram literature between 1937 and 2000 and reviewed 13 clinical trials of disulfiram between the years 2000 and 2008. Disulfiram proved to be an effective therapeutic tool in all studies with superiority being documented in majority of the trials. Initial psychoeducation regarding the mechanism of action of disulfiram and its therapeutic implications are a must for efficacious use of the drug while disulfiram also may be extended to serve as a coping skill for the patient with dependence under treatment [20].

Disulfiram can be a useful option in the long term if given under supervision by a family member where it contributes to longer periods of sobriety in alcohol dependent patients [21]. Another paper speaks about the long-term safety and efficacy of supervised disulfiram and reports a 70% complete abstinence in patients who were maintained on supervised disulfiram. The complete abstinence in the patients was for a mean period of 70.1 ± 23.5 months and the first relapse occurred after a mean of 34.7 ± 15.5 months [22]. Some studies show the successful use of a breath analyzer to assess compliance status of patients on disulfiram. But the cost of a breath analyzer is often a deterrent to its use in small routine clinical settings [23].

There are some shortcomings in the research design and methodology of many disulfiram studies. In a review on outcome studies on disulfiram treatment, it was concluded that only 1 out of more than 40 odd studies between the late 1930s and 1970s met adequate research design criteria [24]. Authors in another paper have found that only of 5 of 135 research studies with disulfiram were controlled clinical trials. This difficulty and other limitations in using valid and reliable study designs have resulted in diverse outcomes in disulfiram research [25]. The main methodological concerns have been a lack of blinding, poor or a lack of measurement of treatment adherence, small follow-up periods, failure to include disulfiram as part of comprehensive treatment and lack of randomization of subjects [26].

Studies with disulfiram have rarely used control groups, and the participants were often not blinded to the treatment groups. The reason behind this was the basic of mechanism of action of disulfiram that entails that subjects need to know that they are on disulfiram for its full effect to occur. The role of the psychological effect or threat of the disulfiram ethanol reaction is an important factor in the efficacy of disulfiram. There is also another thought in disulfiram studies that anyways blinding may easily break when a subject takes a drink and gets a reaction, hence no blinding is appropriate. The problem of unmasking the blind by a medication's side effects is not unique to disulfiram, but the experience of disulfiram–ethanol reaction directly influences outcomes measure, such as increasing abstinence [27].

In the most cited disulfiram study, which had adequate power and blinding, the study was also the first clinical trial on disulfiram to monitor medication adherence to examine its effect on drinking outcomes. 605 of 6629 Veterans Administration inpatient and outpatient treatment patients, who were younger than 60 years and met the National Council on Alcoholism diagnostic criteria for alcoholism, were randomized. There were three conditions viz. disulfiram treatment (250 mg) with 50 mg of riboflavin; blinded disulfiram treatment (250 mg) with 50 mg of riboflavin; and no disulfiram with 50 mg of riboflavin. Riboflavin was added to measure the level of medication adherence. The study's blinded group was an ingenious attempt to expose the participants to the psychological threat of disulfiram–ethanol reaction without the actual pharmacological reaction, thereby making it possible to measure the effectiveness of disulfiram. No significant differences among the three treatment groups in rate of abstinence or 'the time to first drink day' were noted. Across all treatment conditions, the participants who showed a high degree of treatment adherence were the most successful in maintaining abstinence from alcohol and 20% of 577 patients completed the study. Disulfiram-treated patients who attended all seven assessment visits lowered their frequency in drinking as compared with the other study groups suggests that disulfiram can provide benefits to those who are motivated in attending appointments [11].

In a review on disulfiram, authors argue that patients who are adherent with disulfiram essentially approach other treatment regimens in a similarly yielding manner, such that these treatment-adherent patients will be able to achieve long-term abstinence, regardless of whether they are taking disulfiram. In addition, if a patient decides to take disulfiram with the knowledge of the disulfiram–ethanol reactions, the individual is presumably more determined to abstain from drinking [28]. Adherence is a crucial methodological issue in determining the generalization of the effectiveness of disulfiram.

Techniques to enhance treatment adherence, such as supervised disulfiram treatment or incentive-driven interventions, have reportedly shown to be associated with better disulfiram outcomes [29].

A study objectively examining the effectiveness of the supervised disulfiram treatment found that twice-weekly supervised disulfiram treatment significantly enhanced the treatment session attendance and abstinence [30]. Disulfiram supervision as a part of a community reinforcement programme, which included behavioural interventions for psychosocial domains (employment and marital relationship), also showed significantly better results than a standard outpatient programme did in reducing drinking frequency and maintaining abstinence [31].

In a review of published clinical studies using direct supervised disulfiram treatment, the researcher reported that 17 of 18 studies demonstrated positive outcomes. A closer examination of the work reveals that the literature included case studies using descriptive analyses without statistical comparisons, retrospective studies without comparison groups, or randomized controlled trials without adequate power [32].

Many studies of disulfiram efficacy have outcome variables that include non-drinking measures, such as the number of arrests, treatment retention period, work absenteeism, quality of life indicators and postoperative complications and confounding factors commonly accompanied a supervised disulfiram condition, such that the role of supervised disulfiram treatment was often unclear [33].

One study used a randomized assignment and a control showed that supervised disulfiram treatment (200 mg) yielded enhanced treatment outcome when compared with a control group receiving vitamin C. Clinical staff or the spouse of the patients provided daily supervision of medication intake and received support from the clinic about working with patients who refused the medication. Patients in both the supervised disulfiram and the vitamin C group shared similar rates of treatment adherence, but the supervised disulfiram group obtained a significantly higher number of abstinent days and a lower amount of drinks during the 6-month trial. This supports the fact that supervised disulfiram can be a useful tool in managing drinking behaviour for those patients seeking treatment [34].

In a recent single-blinded, randomized placebo-controlled study, 109 patients diagnosed with alcohol dependence under ICD-10 criteria were randomly allocated to four treatment groups, depending on whether they took disulfiram (200 mg daily) or a placebo or whether they received adjunctive therapy consisting of mailed letters which delineated and emphasized the harmful effect of alcohol and the management of alcohol craving. The proportion of abstinence among the four groups at 26 weeks after discharge was the primary outcome measure. The proportion of abstinence was compared with the severity of alcohol dependence and craving. There were no significant differences among the four groups in terms of abstinent patients or study dropouts. The ratio of abstinence was not related to the severity of alcohol dependence or the degree of alcohol craving [35].

In a pharmacogenetic study, alcohol-dependent subjects received naltrexone alone, placebo alone, disulfiram with placebo or disulfiram with naltrexone. They were genotyped for certain genes and 107 male European-American subjects were included in the study. There were no significant interactions of the genes with Naltrexone on the primary outcome of abstinence from heavy drinking. The DBH genotype interacted with disulfiram on drinks per drinking day with less drinking for subjects with the genotype than for T allele carriers on disulfiram [36].

3.3 Disulfiram Implant Therapy

Disulfiram has been used for over four decades as a subcutaneous implantation which was first introduced in 1968. The origin of disulfiram implants was to overcome adherence problems while in most studies the effectiveness of disulfiram implants remains debatable [37]. Researchers examined the effectiveness of disulfiram implants as compared with placebo controls by using sham operations or calcium phosphate implants. In one study, disulfiram implants did not show an advantage over placebo, although the patients in both disulfiram implant and placebo groups achieved a longer duration of abstinence after the treatment when compared with the abstinence duration before the treatment. The longer period of abstinence in both groups after the intervention, when compared with the period before the intervention, demonstrated that disulfiram is a psychological deterrent [38]. Other studies showed that disulfiram implants (800 mg) produced either a significant increase in days of abstinence or a significantly longer abstinence duration when compared with placebo. In these studies, more than 50% of the patients who drank alcohol in disulfiram implant group experienced disulfiram–ethanol reactions after relapsing to drinking, evidencing that the pharmacological effects of disulfiram increased the abstinent duration or days of abstinence [39, 40]. Disulfiram implants were also tested in different doses and showed that the drinking outcomes were not significantly different for three disulfiram implant dose conditions (800, 1200 and 1600 mg) when comparing post-treatment drinking behaviours. This study also demonstrated that the patients in all three conditions drank less during post treatment period than during pre-treatment period, again supporting the psychological deterring effect of disulfiram [41].

Recent disulfiram implant efficacy studies have shown mixed results and have not performed significantly better than placebo in controlled clinical trials. In the most recent randomized, double-blinded, placebo-controlled trial, for example, the patients in the implanted disulfiram and in the placebo implant condition (calcium phosphate) were both led to believe that they were receiving disulfiram implants. The two groups did not significantly differ in drinking measures or the time to first relapse, with both groups reducing their drinking significantly. The findings emphasize that the psychological effect of disulfiram (deterring patients from drinking by informing them of disulfiram–ethanol reaction) rather than the pharmacological effect is the primary therapeutic action of disulfiram [42].

Researchers have asserted that the lack of disulfiram implant efficacy in these trials, when compared with placebo, could be because of the insignificant absorption of disulfiram implant or inadequate amount of disulfiram being released, compared with daily oral dose, as shown by infrequent disulfiram–ethanol reaction reports in many studies. The disulfiram implant patients who experienced disulfiram–ethanol reactions, as subsequently abstained from alcohol or drank less [43]. There are ethical concerns about the pharmacological role of disulfiram by the induction of disulfiram–ethanol reactions and whether this adverse reaction and its consequence should be used to treat alcoholism, a condition with serious medical and psychological consequences [44]. The role of disulfiram implants in the long-term management of alcohol dependence is still debatable and many countries have not approved the use of these implants.

3.4 Do Certain Patients Respond Better to Disulfiram Therapy?

There are studies that have shown subgroups of patients who showed benefits from disulfiram treatment, and a refined list of these patients' characteristics has been further offered [45]. Authors have reviewed the literature covering this theme and suggested that the results are partly contradictory [43]. In general, the patient characteristics associated with better disulfiram treatment outcomes are viz. older individuals (older than 40 years) with longer drinking history, socially stable, high motivation to quit, regular Alcoholics Anonymous attendance, being able to maintain and tolerate dependent or treatment relationships, cognitive intactness and good family support [46]. Further research in focusing on patient factors related to successful outcome with disulfiram therapy would provide general guidelines to select patients for disulfiram treatment who are likely to show optimal effectiveness.

3.5 Points of Clinical Relevance

1. There are mixed reports and reviews on the efficacy of disulfiram in alcohol dependence. While some authors believe that it is among the most successful medications for alcohol dependence, there are others who consider it just another second-line medication with moderate efficacy.
2. Fear of the Disulfiram–Ethanol Reaction (DER) in clinicians and its effects on their patients along with issues related to high cost and lack of easy availability of disulfiram in certain nations may have added to moderation of its use.
3. Clinical experience and personal communications with many psychiatrists have been revealing that lack of exposure to disulfiram use during psychiatry residency and training often serves as a deterrent in its use at a later stage during private clinical practice.
4. There is a need for regular disulfiram use in substance abuse practice across countries due to its deterrent action and high relapse prevention mechanism. There is also a need for disulfiram to be used in diverse patient populations to know its efficacy in various settings.
5. The patient knowing that he is on disulfiram is vital to its action and must be emphasized upon during family and patient psycho-education before the initia-

tion of treatment. This must be repeated during treatment to reinforce the effects of disulfiram at various time periods during the treatment.

6. Many psychiatrists perceive disulfiram as a psychological tool to induce motivation through creating fear of drinking. Failure and success are perceived as related to the level of motivation. These perceptions could be unfair as biological factors in inter-patient variability in response are ignored. These views on the effectiveness and safety of the drug and the necessity of providing stringent even intrusive motivation and monitoring may discourage some practitioners from becoming involved in such interventions.

3.6 Conclusion

Disulfiram is being used successfully for over seven decades now in the long-term management of alcohol dependence. It is one of the oldest molecules used in alcohol dependence pharmacotherapy and has stood the test of time. Since usage of disulfiram needs continued and repeated consultation with the treating psychiatrist and active decision making by the patient, it is likely that such consultations give a chance to both of them to improve the abstinence attempts of the patient. Disulfiram has been extensively studied and well understood over the years. The psychological aspects of supervised disulfiram therapy along with regular consultations with the psychiatrist contribute to a good clinical outcome with the drug in alcohol dependence.

References

1. Koppaka V, Thompson DC, Chen Y, Ellermann M, Nicolaou KC, Juvonen RO, Petersen D, Deitrich RA, Hurley TD, Vasiliou V. Aldehyde dehydrogenase inhibitors: a comprehensive review of the pharmacology, mechanism of action, substrate specificity, and clinical application. Pharmacol Rev. 2012;64(3):520–39.
2. Lipsky JJ, Shen ML, Naylor S. Overview—in vitro inhibition of aldehyde dehydrogenase by disulfiram and metabolites. Chem Biol Interact. 2001;130:81–91.
3. Bourcier S, Mongardon N, Daviaud F, Moachon L, Arnould MA, Perruche F, Pène F, Cariou A. Disulfiram ethanol reaction mimicking anaphylactic, cardiogenic, and septic shock. Am J Emerg Med. 2013;31(1):270–1.
4. Shen ML, Lipsky JJ, Naylor S. Role of disulfiram in the in vitro inhibition of rat liver mitochondrial aldehyde dehydrogenase. Biochem Pharmacol. 2000;60(7):947–53.
5. Kosten TR, Wu G, Huang W, Harding MJ, Hamon SC, Lappalainen J, Nielsen DA. Pharmacogenetic randomized trial for cocaine abuse: disulfiram and dopamine β-hydroxylase. Biol Psychiatry. 2013;73(3):219–24.
6. Jung YC, Namkoong K. Pharmacotherapy for alcohol dependence: anti-craving medications for relapse prevention. Yonsei Med J. 2006;47(2):167–78.
7. Müller CA, Banas R. Disulfiram: an anti-craving substance? Am J Psychiatry. 2011;168(1):98–102.
8. Johnson BA, Mann K, Willenbring ML, Litten RZ, Swift RM, Lesch OM, Berglund M. Challenges and opportunities for medications development in alcoholism: an interna-

tional perspective on collaborations between academia and industry. Alcohol Clin Exp Res. 2005;29(8):1528–40.
9. Skinner MD, Lahmek P, Pham H, Aubin HJ. Disulfiram efficacy in the treatment of alcohol dependence: a meta-analysis. PLoS One. 2014;9(2):e87366.
10. Ulrichsen J, Nielsen MK, Ulrichsen M. Disulfiram in severe alcoholism—an open controlled study. Nord J Psychiatry. 2010;64(6):356–62.
11. Fuller RK, Branchey L, Brightwell DR, Derman RM, Emrick CD, Iber FL, James KE, Lacoursiere RB, Lee KK, Lowenstam I, Maany I. Disulfiram treatment of alcoholism: a veterans administration cooperative study. JAMA. 1986;256(11):1449–55.
12. Brewer C. Recent developments in disulfiram treatment. Alcohol Alcohol. 1993;28(4):383–95.
13. Børup C, Kaiser A, Jensen E. Long-term Antabuse treatment: tolerance and reasons for withdraw-al. Acta Psychiatr Scand. 1992;86:47–9.
14. Liskow B, Nickel E, Tunley N, Powell B, Penick EE. Alcoholics' attitudes toward and experiences with disulfiram. Am J Drug Alcohol Abuse. 1990;16(1–2):147–60.
15. Brewer C, Meyers RJ, Johnsen J. Does disulfiram help to prevent relapse in alcohol abuse? CNS Drugs. 2000;14(5):329–41.
16. Brewer C. Long-term, high-dose disulfiram in the treatment of alcohol abuse. Br J Psychiatry. 1993;163(5):687–9.
17. Mutschler J, Dirican G, Funke S, Obermann C, Grosshans M, Mann K, Kiefer F, Diehl A. Experienced acetaldehyde reaction does not improve treatment response in outpatients treated with supervised disulfiram. Clin Neuropharmacol. 2011;34(4):161–5.
18. Krampe H, Stawicki S, Hoehe MR, Ehrenreich H. Outpatient Long-term Intensive Therapy for Alcoholics (OLITA): a successful biopsychosocial approach to the treatment of alcoholism. Dialogues Clin Neurosci. 2007;9(4):399–412.
19. Krampe H, Ehrenreich H. Supervised disulfiram as adjunct to psychotherapy in alcoholism treatment. Curr Pharm Des. 2010;16(19):2076–90.
20. Suh JJ, Pettinati HM, Kampman KM, O'Brien CP. The status of disulfiram: a half of a century later. J Clin Psychopharmacol. 2006;26(3):290–302.
21. Mutschler J, Dirican G, Gutzeit A, Grosshans M. Safety and efficacy of long-term disulfiram aftercare. Clin Neuropharmacol. 2011;34(5):195–8.
22. Mutschler J, Diehl A, Kiefer F. Pharmacology of disulfiram—an update. Fortschr Neurol Psychiatr. 2008;76(4):225–31.
23. Fletcher K, Stone E, Mohamad MW, Faulder GC, Faulder RM, Jones K, Morgan D, Wegerdt J, Kelly M, Chick J. A breath test to assess compliance with disulfiram. Addiction. 2006;101(12):1705–10.
24. Baekeland F, Lundwall L, Kissin B, Shanahan T. Correlates of outcome in disulfiram treatment of alcoholism. J Nerv Ment Dis. 1971;153(1):1–9.
25. Garbutt JC. The state of pharmacotherapy for the treatment of alcohol dependence. J Subst Abuse Treat. 2009;36(1):S15–23.
26. Garbutt JC, West SL, Carey TS, Lohr KN, Crews FT. Pharmacological treatment of alcohol dependence: a review of the evidence. JAMA. 1999;281(14):1318–25.
27. Kalra G, De Sousa A, Shrivastava A. Disulfiram in the management of alcohol dependence: a comprehensive clinical review. Open J Psychiatry. 2014;4(1):43.
28. Banys P. The clinical use of disulfiram (Antabuse®): a review. J Psychoactive Drugs. 1988;20(3):243–61.
29. De Sousa A. The pharmacotherapy of alcohol dependence: a state of the art review. Mens Sana Monogr. 2010;8(1):69–82.
30. Gerrein JR, Rosenberg CM, Manohar V. Disulfiram maintenance in outpatient treatment of alcoholism. Arch Gen Psychiatry. 1973;28:799–802.
31. Azrin NH. Improvements in the community-reinforcement approach to alcoholism. Behav Res Ther. 1976;14:339–48.
32. Brewer C. Supervised disulfiram in alcoholism. Br J Hosp Med. 1986;35(2):116–8.
33. O'Shea B. Disulfiram revisited. Hosp Med. 2000;61(12):849–51.

34. Chick J, Gough K, Falkowski W, Kershaw P, Hore B, Mehta B, Ritson B, Ropner R, Torley D. Disulfiram treatment of alcoholism. Br J Psychiatry. 1992;161(1):84–9.
35. Yoshimura A, Kimura M, Nakayama H, Matsui T, Okudaira F, Akazawa S, Ohkawara M, Cho T, Kono Y, Hashimoto K, Kumagai M. Efficacy of disulfiram for the treatment of alcohol dependence assessed with a multicenter randomized controlled trial. Alcohol Clin Exp Res. 2014;38(2):572–8.
36. Arias AJ, Gelernter J, Gueorguieva R, Ralevski E, Petrakis IL. Pharmacogenetics of naltrexone and disulfiram in alcohol dependent, dually diagnosed veterans. Am J Addict. 2014;23(3):288–93.
37. Allen JP, Litten RZ. Techniques to enhance compliance with disulfiram. Alcohol Clin Exp Res. 1992;16(6):1035–41.
38. Wilson A, Davidson WJ, Blanchard R. Disulfiram implantation: a trial using placebo implants and two types of controls. J Stud Alcohol. 1980;41(5):429–36.
39. Wilson A, Davidson WJ, Blanchard R, White J. Disulfiram implantation. A placebo-controlled trial with two-year follow-up. J Stud Alcohol. 1978;39(5):809–19.
40. Wilson A. Disulfiram implantation in alcoholism treatment. A review. J Stud Alcohol. 1975;36(5):555–65.
41. Wilson A, Davidson WJ, White J. Disulfiram implantation: placebo, psychological deterrent, and pharmacological deterrent effects. Br J Psychiatry. 1976;129(3):277–80.
42. Johnsen J, Mørland J. Depot preparations of disulfiram: experimental and clinical results. Acta Psychiatr Scand. 1992;86(S369):27–30.
43. Hughes JC, Cook CC. The efficacy of disulfiram: a review of outcome studies. Addiction. 1997;92(4):381–95.
44. Barth KS, Malcolm RJ. Disulfiram: an old therapeutic with new applications. CNS Neurol Disord Drug Targets. 2010;9(1):5–12.
45. Fuller RK, Gordis E. Does disulfiram have a role in alcoholism treatment today? Addiction. 2004;99(1):21–4.
46. Jørgensen CH, Pedersen B, Tønnesen H. The efficacy of disulfiram for the treatment of alcohol use disorder. Alcohol Clin Exp Res. 2011;35(10):1749–58.

Disulfiram in the Management of Cocaine Dependence and Other Psychiatric Disorders

4

4.1 Introduction

Cocaine dependence and abuse is one of the growing substance use problems in the world today. There has been a rise in the number of cocaine users in the world exponentially in the last decade [1]. Cocaine is also a preferred drug of use because it has very few physical withdrawal symptoms and most of the withdrawal symptoms are psychological in nature which can be managed well with medications [2]. Despite decades of significant advances in the understanding of the actions of cocaine on neural chemistry, an effective medical treatment for cocaine dependence has remained elusive [3]. Over the years there have been reports that disulfiram, which is presently indicated for the treatment of alcohol dependence, has shown potential as a treatment for cocaine dependence in most randomized clinical trials and case series [4]. The present chapter looks at various studies of disulfiram in cocaine dependence and tries establishing its true position in the management of the disorder.

4.2 Mechanism of Action of Disulfiram in Cocaine Dependence

Disulfiram has several mechanisms of action. Among these, disulfiram's metabolite, diethyldithiocarbamate, chelates copper and thereby inhibits many copper-dependent enzymes, including dopamine b-hydroxylase (DBH) [5]. This enzyme catalyzes the conversion of dopamine (DA) to norepinephrine (NE) [6] (Fig. 4.1). Inhibition of DBH increases brain levels of DA and decreases the synthesis of NE in animals and humans [7, 8].

Disulfiram treatment also inhibits aldehyde dehydrogenase (ALDH) by a non-copper-dependent mechanism [9]. Alcohol is normally metabolized to acetaldehyde, which ALDH metabolizes to acetic acid. ALDH inhibition leads to the buildup of high levels of acetaldehyde after alcohol consumption causing the

A. De Sousa, *Disulfiram*, https://doi.org/10.1007/978-981-32-9876-7_4

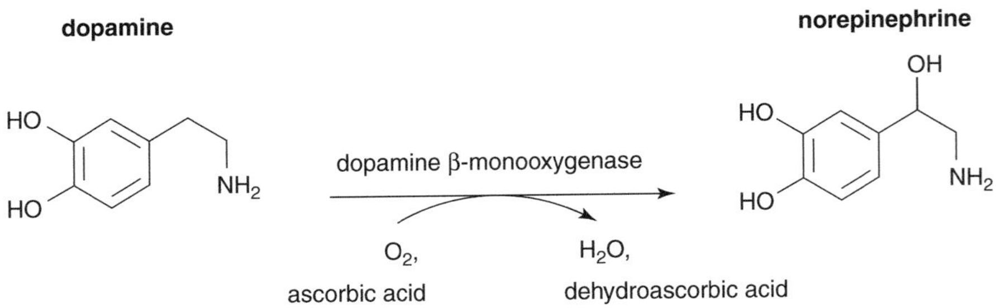

Fig. 4.1 Dopamine metabolism

flushing, nausea, uneasiness, hypotension and vomiting characterizing the disulfiram–alcohol reaction [10]. This reaction (or fear of this reaction) is thought to be the mechanism responsible for disulfiram's efficacy in the treatment of alcohol dependence [11].

In addition, disulfiram inhibits carboxylesterase and cholinesterase by unknown mechanisms [12]. This reduces the metabolism of cocaine, increasing plasma levels of cocaine, which may then cause its cardiovascular effects [13]. In addition to the inhibition of the dopamine transporter (DAT) [14] cocaine also inhibits the norepinephrine and serotonin transporters (NET and SERT), increasing synaptic levels of all three neurotransmitters [15]. Cocaine-induced increase in synaptic DA is a cause of its substance abuse and reinforcing effects [16], though recent research suggests that NE also plays an important role in the same [17]. Clinical studies evaluating the impact of disulfiram treatment have produced three types of results, where it has been shown that disulfiram decreases cocaine's positive subjective effects [18] or increases some of its negative effects such as anxiety and paranoia [19] or produces no changes at all in some patients [20].

The efficacy of disulfiram in treating cocaine dependence has been attributed to several different mechanisms, including a decrease in cocaine reward mechanisms, an increase in cocaine aversion, and/or as a 'DA replacement therapy' that elevates DA levels and restores normal reward function in hypodopaminergic addicts [21, 22]. DBH inhibition has been suggested to underlie disulfiram's efficacy in cocaine dependence but this hypothesis has not been tested directly (Fig. 4.2) [23].

4.3 Disulfiram in Cocaine Dependence—A Review of Studies Done

In the last years the interest in the use of disulfiram for the treatment of cocaine dependence has increased consistently. Both preclinical and clinical studies have investigated the potential efficacy of disulfiram for this substance use disorder, the neurobiological bases for its effect and related safety issues [24].

The initial reasons for the use of disulfiram to treat cocaine dependence was the high rate of comorbidity between cocaine abuse or dependence and alcohol abuse or

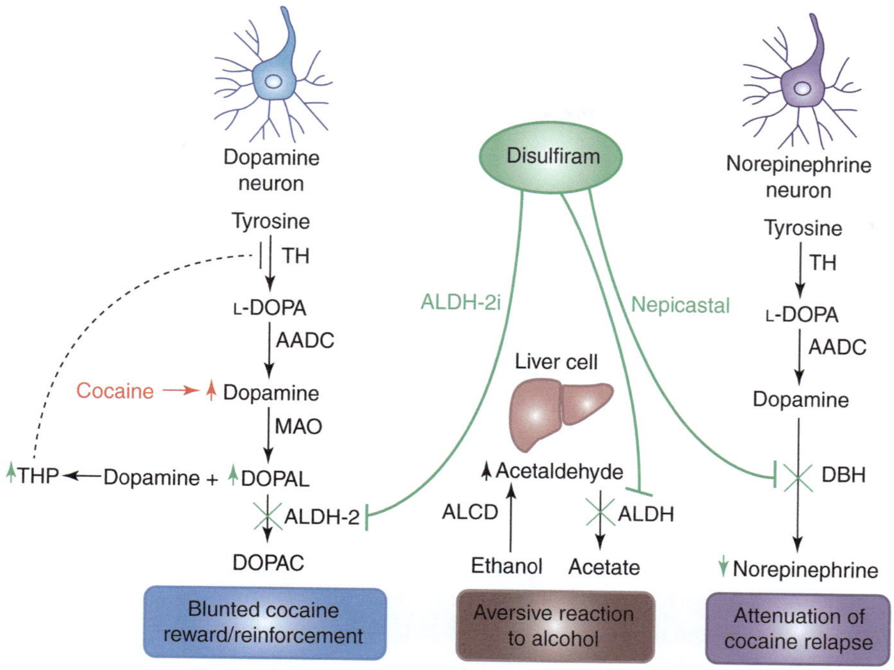

Fig. 4.2 Effect of Disulfiram on Dopamine metabolism. (Free for use from https://www.tumblr.com/tagged/antabuse)

dependence, up to 60–85% in certain studies [25]. The theory posited was that a reduction in alcohol use would lead to secondary reduction in cocaine use. The abstinence from alcohol would also prevent formation of cocaethylene, a metabolite formed when alcohol and cocaine are present together. Cocaethylene has pharmacological actions similar to cocaine, but may be longer acting [26].

A recent 12-week open-labelled study in outpatients abusing both cocaine and alcohol found that the four patients receiving disulfiram (400 mg/day) along with CBT had fewer urine samples positive for cocaine than patients receiving CBT alone [27].

In an early randomized controlled trial in 122 combined cocaine–alcohol substance abusers it was noted that disulfiram treatment was associated with significantly better retention in treatment, as well as longer duration of abstinence from alcohol and cocaine use. The two active psychotherapies (cognitive behaviour therapy and 12-step facilitation) were associated with reduced cocaine use over time compared with supportive psychotherapy. Cocaine and alcohol use were strongly related throughout treatment, particularly for subjects treated with disulfiram. Disulfiram combined with outpatient psychotherapy was thus considered a promising treatment strategy for cocaine users [28].

In another randomized controlled trial, the study was designed to compare the effectiveness of disulfiram therapy with that of a placebo condition in reducing cocaine use and to compare the effectiveness of two active behavioural therapies—cognitive behavior therapy (CBT) and interpersonal psychotherapy (IPT)—in reducing cocaine use. It was noted that when 121 subjects enrolled for the study, participants assigned to disulfiram reduced their cocaine use significantly more than those assigned to placebo, and those assigned to CBT reduced their cocaine use significantly more than those assigned to IPT. Benefits of disulfiram use and CBT were most pronounced for participants who were not alcohol dependent at baseline or who fully abstained from drinking alcohol during treatment [29].

In a study on disulfiram for the management of cocaine dependence in patients with comorbid opioid dependence, 67 cocaine-dependent, methadone-maintained, opioid-dependent subjects were given either disulfiram or placebo. Disulfiram-treated subjects decreased the quantity and frequency of cocaine use significantly more than those treated with placebo. Alcohol use was minimal for all subjects regardless of the medication. Thus it was concluded that disulfiram may be an effective pharmacotherapy for cocaine abuse among methadone-maintained opioid addicts, even in those individuals without comorbid alcohol abuse [30].

In a long-term 1-year follow-up study of 96 patients it has been noted that, as a group, participants reported significant decreases in frequency of cocaine, but not alcohol use, after the end of treatment. Secondly, the main effects of disulfiram on cocaine and alcohol use were sustained during follow-up. Finally, initiation of abstinence for even brief periods of time within treatment was associated with significantly better outcome during follow-up. This indicates that disulfiram has a potential role in the long-term management of cocaine dependence [31]. In another study on 20 subjects with combined opioid and cocaine dependence, the subjects were induced onto buprenorphine maintenance and then randomized to disulfiram (250 mg) treatment for 12 weeks. Fifteen subjects completed the study, including eight subjects randomized to disulfiram (72.7%) and seven subjects randomized to placebo (77.8%). The total number of weeks abstinent from cocaine was significantly greater on disulfiram versus placebo and the number of days to achieving 3 weeks of continuous cocaine abstinence was significantly lower in disulfiram compared with placebo. The number of cocaine-negative urine tests during the trial was also higher on disulfiram than on placebo. Furthermore, subjects in the disulfiram group achieved consistently higher rates of cocaine-negative urine tests in each 3-week interval and the increase over time was faster in the disulfiram compared with placebo [32]. In another study on 161 methadone-maintained opioid and cocaine abusers, disulfiram has shown efficacy in the successful abstinence from cocaine abuse [33]. In an early pilot study, 18 outpatients dependent on both cocaine and alcohol were randomly assigned to disulfiram or naltrexone in an open pilot study. Disulfiram treatment resulted in significantly fewer days of alcohol and cocaine use, with longer sustained periods of abstinence from both substances [34].

In a recent study, 208 patients were randomized to disulfiram (250 mg/day), naltrexone (100 mg/day), the combination, or placebo for 11 weeks. Outcomes were in-trial abstinence from cocaine and/or alcohol. Abstinence from cocaine as measured by cocaine-negative urines and days of self-reported abstinence from cocaine or alcohol did not differ between placebo and any of the medication groups. However, patients taking disulfiram (alone or in combination) were most likely to achieve combined abstinence from cocaine and alcohol. Secondary analyses revealed that patients taking the disulfiram–naltrexone combination were most likely to achieve 3 consecutive weeks of abstinence from cocaine and alcohol [35].

Studies have also looked at sex-based differences in disulfiram for the management of cocaine dependence. Sex-by-treatment interactions from two pooled randomized clinical trials involving 191 cocaine-dependent subjects (36% female) were evaluated. Primary outcomes were days of abstinence and percentage of drug-free urine specimens. Significant sex-by-treatment interactions were found, where men treated with disulfiram had better outcomes than those who were not. Women had an intermediate outcome regardless of whether they received disulfiram. Sex differences in response to disulfiram treatment have important clinical and theoretical implications and are worthy of further study [36].

Several short-term clinical trials in outpatients using both cocaine and alcohol showed that disulfiram (250–500 mg/day), along with CBT or a 12-step self-help group, significantly reduced cocaine and alcohol use [37]. In human laboratory studies, disulfiram inhibits cocaine metabolism, increasing cocaine plasma levels when the two are administered together. In some studies, this has been associated with enhanced cardiovascular response to cocaine. Both cocaine and the disulfiram–alcohol interaction can produce severe cardiovascular effects. A patient who relapsed to cocaine and/or alcohol use while taking disulfiram might be at risk for serious, perhaps life-threatening, adverse events. This might limit the use of disulfiram to patients who are highly motivated for abstinence, have an active social support network for early detection of relapse, and are in good cardiovascular health [38].

In a recent study on 112 methadone-maintenance subjects that received disulfiram, it was noted that assignment to 12 step-facilitation was associated with less cocaine use throughout treatment and a higher number of cocaine-negative urines. While there were no significant main effects of disulfiram versus placebo, individuals without an alcohol use disorder demonstrated greater reductions in cocaine use over time when assigned to disulfiram [39]. In a recent factorial randomized double blind (for medication condition) clinical trial, cognitive behavioural therapy (CBT) served as the platform and was delivered in weekly individual sessions in a community-based outpatient clinic. Ninety-nine outpatients who met DSM-IV criteria for current cocaine dependence were assigned to receive either disulfiram or placebo with or without contingency management (CM). The primary hypothesis that CM and disulfiram would produce the best cocaine outcomes was not confirmed, nor was there a main effect for disulfiram. For the primary outcome (percent days of abstinence, self report), there was a significant interaction, with the best cocaine outcomes were seen for the combination of CM and placebo, with the two groups assigned to disulfiram associated with intermediate outcomes, and poorest cocaine outcome among those assigned to placebo and no CM. CM enhances outcomes for CBT treatment of cocaine dependence, but disulfiram provided no added benefit to the combination of CM and CBT in this study [40].

In another study on 434 subjects from various clinical trials when gender differences were evaluated, it was noted that women, compared with men, had poorer treatment outcomes on multiple measures of cocaine use during treatment and at post-treatment follow-up. These results appear to be primarily accounted for by disulfiram being less effective in women compared with men. There was no evidence of meaningful gender differences in outcome as a function of the behavioural therapies evaluated [41].

In a cost-effectiveness study of disulfiram it was shown in 67 cocaine-dependent methadone-maintained opioid-dependent subjects who were randomized to get the additional treatment of disulfiram or placebo in a 12-week trial, that even though disulfiram increases slightly the cost of methadone treatment, its increase in effectiveness may be important enough to warrant its addition for treating cocaine dependence in methadone-maintained opiate addicts [42].

In another study, 17 non-treatment seeking, cocaine-dependent volunteers participated in this double-blind, placebo-controlled, laboratory-based study. A cross-over design was utilized in which participants received placebo in one phase and disulfiram (250 mg/day) in the other. Following 3 days of study medication participants completed two choice sessions. In one they made ten choices between receiving an intravenous infusion of saline or money that increased in value and in the other cocaine (20 mg) or money. Participants chose cocaine more than saline under both disulfiram and placebo conditions. Unexpectedly, disulfiram increased both the number of cocaine and saline infusion choices. Disulfiram dose (mg/kg bodyweight) was negatively correlated with number of choices for cocaine and disulfiram also enhanced cocaine-induced increases in cardiovascular measures [43].

In a Cochrane database review of disulfiram in the management of cocaine dependence, seven studies with 492 participants met the inclusion criteria for the review. There were no statistically significant results for dropouts but a trend favouring disulfiram when compared to placebo. For cocaine use, it was not possible to pool together primary studies, results from single studies showed that, one, out of four comparisons, was in favour of disulfiram. When disulfiram versus no pharmacological treatment for cocaine use was evaluated a statistically significant difference in favour of disulfiram was noted. The review concluded that there is low evidence, at the present, supporting the clinical use of disulfiram for the treatment of cocaine dependence and larger randomized investigations are needed investigating relevant outcomes and reporting data to allow comparisons of results between studies [44].

4.4 Some Other Hypotheses on the Mechanism of Action of Disulfiram in Cocaine Dependence

Laboratory studies have been carried out to understand how disulfiram treatment affects an individual's response to cocaine, and to shed light on the mechanism driving the reduction in cocaine intake. The results have been conflicting across studies. There have been reports of a non-significant increase in 'high' and 'anxiety', whereas others found increases in nervousness, paranoia or psychosis [45, 46]. Other side effects of disulfiram clinical trials on cocaine dependence are headaches, fatigue and paranoia [47]. Thus, there may be a disulfiram–cocaine reaction that is similar to but yet different from the disulfiram–ethanol reaction and that probably promotes cocaine abstinence.

In animal studies, disulfiram has minimal effects on baseline activity levels, but repeated administration prior to cocaine facilitates the development of behavioural sensitization to cocaine in rats [48] and disulfiram pretreatment also enhances cocaine-induced seizures in mice [8].

There is a relationship between dopamine and glutamate in learning and memory and recent research has focused on dopamine–glutamate interactions in the modulation of psychostimulant-induced synaptic plasticity and addiction [49]. Glutamate receptor modulation has potential roles in the behavioural responses to psychostimulants in animal models of addiction [50]. The effects of disulfiram on glutamatergic neurotransmission are not well characterized and the animal study evidence is insufficient to hypothesize a glutamate-related mechanism of action [51].

4.5 Disulfiram and Its Potential Role in the Management of Pathological Gambling

Pathological gambling (PG) is a disorder characterized by recurrent and pathological patterns of gambling associated with a range of social and psychological problems like high rates of bankruptcy, divorce, suicide and reduced quality of life [52]. Comorbidity in PG maybe 34–80% for substance use disorders (excluding tobacco) [53] and is three times higher than in the general population for patients with alcohol dependence [53]. There are probable common pathophysiological factors that might underlie PG and drug addiction, which remain to be proven. PG was considered to be initially an impulse control disorder and has now been included under substance use disorders in DSM-5 [54, 55]. The similarities between PG and drug dependence include not only phenomenological criteria but also epidemiological, clinical, genetic and neurobiological characteristics [56].

There are similar brain structures and neural circuits involved in PG and drug addiction.

Reduced activity in the ventral striatum and the ventromedial and ventrolateral prefrontal cortex has been reported in PG, which is also a hallmark of drug addiction [57]. Elevated dopamine levels in problem gamblers is more than in healthy controls which is also similar to substance abusers [58]. It has been suggested that PG might be related to a deficiency of the mesocorticolimbic dopaminergic reward system, as has been shown for drug addiction [59]. The inferior frontal gyrus, which is critically involved in response inhibition and might be particularly impacted by the brain's noradrenergic system, has been shown to play role in PG [60].

The similarities between PG and drug addiction suggest that patients with pathological gambling may also benefit from medication used for the treatment of drug addiction. Pharmacotherapy research and treatment options for PG are limited with few trials available on the same. There is some evidence to suggest that Naltrexone [61], Nacetyl-cysteine [62], Lithium [63] and selective serotonin reuptake inhibitors have some pharmacological role in the management of PG [64].

Disulfiram reduces cocaine craving by increasing neurotransmitter levels of dopamine and decreasing the norepinephrine levels by blocking the activity of the enzyme dopamine beta hydroxylase (DBH) involved in the metabolism of brain monoamines. As similar neurochemical disturbances have been reported in PG, disulfiram might not only be effective in the treatment of cocaine addiction but also in the treatment of PG [65, 66].

There is just one case report where disulfiram has been shown to be efficacious in the management of comorbid alcohol dependence and PG [67]. According to the case report, the patient had abstained from alcohol consumption for >12 months and had not gambled either since treatment with disulfiram was started. One possible explanation might be that the patient was abstinent from alcohol. Furthermore, despite numerous previous detoxifications, the patient had never been treated with supervised disulfiram before and only now was a combined benefit for PG and alcohol observed. Psychological aspects of the supervised disulfiram therapy and the high placebo response rate seen in treatment studies of pathological gambling may have contributed to the good clinical outcome [67]. There is a possible neurobiological contributory factor that disulfiram modulates levels of the brain chemical dopamine and decreasing the norepinephrine levels through blocking the activity of the DBH, which metabolizes brain monoamines. The disappearance of the patient's desire to gamble during treatment with disulfiram points towards the potential of disulfiram in reward modulation in PG, similar to that described in the treatment of cocaine dependence [65, 66]. Larger studies investigating the potential of combined treatment approaches using disulfiram and cognitive behavioural therapies are necessary for PG and disulfiram may be a promising agent to try in the management of PG.

4.6 Some Points of Clinical Relevance

1. Currently, there is little direct evidence supporting an effect of disulfiram on relapse prevention, as most clinical trials have focused on its effect on current cocaine use.
2. Future clinical studies include interviews with participants and objective quantifiable measures that can help distinguish between abstinence due to altered drug effects and the effect of environmental triggers.
3. Disulfiram has been used as an alcohol deterrent agent for decades and recent studies indicate that it is also an effective pharmacotherapy for the treatment of cocaine dependence; however, the mechanisms behind its efficacy for alcohol and for cocaine addiction are different. Whereas aldehyde dehydrogenase is the primary target in treating alcoholism, human and preclinical animal studies have indicated that the beneficial effects of disulfiram in cocaine dependence are a result of the inhibition of DBH. The major effect of disulfiram arises via

the effect of disulfiram-mediated DBH inhibition on cocaine reward reduction and reducing relapse more so the relapse precipitated by stress.
4. The effect of acute and chronic disulfiram treatment on several aspects of dopamine transmission, such as neurochemical and behavioural responses to psychostimulants, need further scientific investigation.
5. The effects of disulfiram on stress-induced, cue induced and drug primed reinstatement of cocaine seeking, as well as the brain regions critical for these effects need to be investigated in large controlled studies.
6. Disulfiram as a treatment for dependence on psychostimulants other than cocaine like amphetamines also warrants research.
7. The study of pharmacogenetic interactions between disulfiram and the DBH genotype shall also yield valuable information.
8. We are very sure that the gains acquired by studying disulfiram further could be translated into the development of safer and better pharmacotherapies for the treatment of cocaine dependence.
9. It is also important to understand that the subject needs to know he is on disulfiram for its effects to happen. Disulfiram may also be limited by its own effects on the liver and other side effects.
10. The effects of disulfiram in different subtypes of cocaine-dependent patients ranging from recreational users to chronic users and with varying comorbidities need further investigation in randomized controlled trials.

4.7 Conclusion

The research on the use of disulfiram in the management of cocaine dependence and pathological gambling is still in a nascent stage with many parameters of the drug in cocaine dependence and its efficacy in subtypes of cocaine dependence yet to be investigated. The use of disulfiram in pathological gambling is limited to case reports and case series and definitely needs further evidence before implementation.

References

1. Calabria B, Degenhardt L, Briegleb C, Vos T, Hall W, Lynskey M, Callaghan B, Rana U, McLaren J. Systematic review of prospective studies investigating remission from amphetamine, cannabis, cocaine or opioid dependence. Addict Behav. 2010;35(8):741–9.
2. Chen CY, Anthony JC. Epidemiological estimates of risk in the process of becoming dependent upon cocaine: cocaine hydrochloride powder versus crack cocaine. Psychopharmacology. 2004;172(1):78–86.
3. Lima MS, Soares BG, Reisser AA, Farrell M. Pharmacological treatment of cocaine dependence: a systematic review. Addiction. 2002;97(8):931–49.
4. Karila L, Gorelick D, Weinstein A, Noble F, Benyamina A, Coscas S, Blecha L, Lowenstein W, Martinot JL, Reynaud M, Lépine JP. New treatments for cocaine dependence: a focused review. Int J Neuropsychopharmacol. 2008;11(3):425–38.
5. Dackis CA, Gold MS. New concepts in cocaine addiction: the dopamine depletion hypothesis. Neurosci Biobehav Rev. 1985;9(3):469–77.

6. Schroeder JP, Cooper DA, Schank JR, Lyle MA, Gaval-Cruz M, Ogbonmwan YE, Pozdeyev N, Freeman KG, Iuvone PM, Edwards GL, Holmes PV. Disulfiram attenuates drug-primed reinstatement of cocaine seeking via inhibition of dopamine β-hydroxylase. Neuropsychopharmacology. 2010;35(12):2440–6.
7. Kosten TR, Wu G, Huang W, Harding MJ, Hamon SC, Lappalainen J, Nielsen DA. Pharmacogenetic randomized trial for cocaine abuse: disulfiram and dopamine β-hydroxylase. Biol Psychiatry. 2013;73(3):219–24.
8. Gaval-Cruz M, Schroeder JP, Liles LC, Javors MA, Weinshenker D. Effects of disulfiram and dopamine beta-hydroxylase knockout on cocaine-induced seizures. Pharmacol Biochem Behav. 2008;89(4):556–62.
9. Suh JJ, Pettinati HM, Kampman KM, O'Brien CP. The status of disulfiram: a half of a century later. J Clin Psychopharmacol. 2006;26(3):290–302.
10. Savas MC, Güllü İH. Disulfiram–ethanol test reaction: significance of supervision. Ann Pharmacother. 1997;31(3):374–5.
11. Krampe H, Ehrenreich H. Supervised disulfiram as adjunct to psychotherapy in alcoholism treatment. Curr Pharm Des. 2010;16(19):2076–90.
12. Savolainen K, Hervonen H, Lehto VP, Mattila MJ. Neurotoxic effects of disulfiram on autonomic nervous system in rat. Acta Pharmacol Toxicol. 1984;55(5):339–44.
13. McCance-Katz EF, Kosten TR, Jatlow P. Chronic disulfiram treatment effects on intranasal cocaine administration: initial results. Biol Psychiatry. 1998;43(7):540–3.
14. Devoto P, Flore G, Saba P, Cadeddu R, Gessa GL. Disulfiram stimulates dopamine release from noradrenergic terminals and potentiates cocaine-induced dopamine release in the prefrontal cortex. Psychopharmacology. 2012;219(4):1153–64.
15. Beck O, Helander A, Carlsson S, Borg S. Changes in serotonin metabolism during treatment with the aldehyde dehydrogenase inhibitors disulfiram and cyanamide. Pharmacol Toxicol. 1995;77(5):323–6.
16. Noble EP. Addiction and its reward process through polymorphisms of the D2 dopamine receptor gene: a review. Eur Psychiatry. 2000;15(2):79–89.
17. Groman SM, James AS, Jentsch JD. Poor response inhibition: at the nexus between substance abuse and attention deficit/hyperactivity disorder. Neurosci Biobehav Rev. 2009;33(5): 690–8.
18. Kalivas PW. Neurobiology of cocaine addiction: implications for new pharmacotherapy. Am J Addict. 2007;16(2):71–8.
19. Hameedi FA, Rosen MI, McCance-Katz EF, McMahon TJ, Price LH, Jatlow PI, Woods SW, Kosten TR. Behavioral, physiological, and pharmacological interaction of cocaine and disulfiram in humans. Biol Psychiatry. 1995;37(8):560–3.
20. Mooney M, Sofuoglu M, Dudish-Poulsen S, Hatsukami DK. Preliminary observations of paranoia in a human laboratory study of cocaine. Addict Behav. 2006;31(7):1245–51.
21. Gaval-Cruz M, Weinshenker D. Mechanisms of disulfiram-induced cocaine abstinence: antabuse and cocaine relapse. Mol Interv. 2009;9(4):175–87.
22. Penberthy JK, Ait-Daoud N, Vaughan M, Fanning T. Review of treatment for cocaine dependence. Curr Drug Abuse Rev. 2010;3(1):49–62.
23. Vocci FJ, Elkashef A. Pharmacotherapy and other treatments for cocaine abuse and dependence. Curr Opin Psychiatry. 2005;18(3):265–70.
24. Shorter D, Domingo CB, Kosten TR. Emerging drugs for the treatment of cocaine use disorder: a review of neurobiological targets and pharmacotherapy. Expert Opin Emerg Drugs. 2015;20(1):15–29.
25. Magura S, Rosenblum A. Modulating effect of alcohol use on cocaine use. Addict Behav. 2000;25(1):117–22.
26. Grassi MC, Cioce AM, Dei Giudici F, Antonilli L, Nencini P. Short-term efficacy of disulfiram or naltrexone in reducing positive urinalysis for both cocaine and cocaethylene in cocaine abusers: a pilot study. Pharmacol Res. 2007;55(2):117–21.
27. Gossop M, Carroll KM. Disulfiram cocaine and alcohol: two outcomes for the price of one? Alcohol Alcohol. 2006;41(2):119–20.

28. Carroll KM, Nich C, Ball SA, McCance E, Rounsavile BJ. Treatment of cocaine and alcohol dependence with psychotherapy and disulfiram. Addiction. 1998;93(5):713–27.
29. Carroll KM, Fenton LR, Ball SA, Nich C, Frankforter TL, Shi J, Rounsaville BJ. Efficacy of disulfiram and cognitive behavior therapy in cocaine-dependent outpatients: a randomized placebo-controlled trial. Arch Gen Psychiatry. 2004;61(3):264–72.
30. Petrakis IL, Carroll KM, Nich C, Gordon LT, McCance-Katz EF, Frankforter T, Rounsaville BJ. Disulfiram treatment for cocaine dependence in methadone-maintained opioid addicts. Addiction. 2000;95(2):219–28.
31. Carroll KM, Nich C, Ball SA, McCance E, Frankforter TL, Rounsaville BJ. One-year follow-up of disulfiram and psychotherapy for cocaine-alcohol users: sustained effects of treatment. Addiction. 2000;95(9):1335–49.
32. George TP, Chawarski MC, Pakes J, Carroll KM, Kosten TR, Schottenfeld RS. Disulfiram versus placebo for cocaine dependence in buprenorphine-maintained subjects: a preliminary trial. Biol Psychiatry. 2000;47(12):1080–6.
33. Oliveto A, Poling J, Mancino MJ, Feldman Z, Cubells JF, Pruzinsky R, Gonsai K, Cargile C, Sofuoglu M, Chopra MP, Gonzalez-Haddad G. Randomized, double blind, placebo-controlled trial of disulfiram for the treatment of cocaine dependence in methadone-stabilized patients. Drug Alcohol Depend. 2011;113(2–3):184–91.
34. Carroll K, Ziedonis D, O'Malley S, McCance-Katz E, Gordon L, Rounsaville B. Pharmacologic interventions for alcohol-and cocaine-abusing individuals: a pilot study of disulfiram vs. naltrexone. Am J Addict. 1993;2(1):77–9.
35. Pettinati HM, Kampman KM, Lynch KG, Xie H, Dackis C, Rabinowitz AR, Charles PO. A double blind, placebo-controlled trial that combines disulfiram and naltrexone for treating co-occurring cocaine and alcohol dependence. Addict Behav. 2008;33(5):651–67.
36. Nich C, McCance-Katz EF, Petrakis IL, Cubells JF, Rounsaville BJ, Carroll KM. Sex differences in cocaine-dependent individuals' response to disulfiram treatment. Addict Behav. 2004;29(6):1123–8.
37. Higgins ST, Budney AJ, Bickel WK, Hughes JR, Foerg F. Disulfiram therapy in patients abusing cocaine and alcohol. Am J Psychiatry. 1993;150(4):675–6.
38. Baker JR, Jatlow P, McCance-Katz EF. Disulfiram effects on responses to intravenous cocaine administration. Drug Alcohol Depend. 2007;87(2–3):202–9.
39. Carroll KM, Nich C, Shi JM, Eagan D, Ball SA. Efficacy of disulfiram and twelve step facilitation in cocaine-dependent individuals maintained on methadone: a randomized placebo-controlled trial. Drug Alcohol Depend. 2012;126(1–2):224–31.
40. Carroll KM, Nich C, Petry NM, Eagan DA, Shi JM, Ball SA. A randomized factorial trial of disulfiram and contingency management to enhance cognitive behavioral therapy for cocaine dependence. Drug Alcohol Depend. 2016;160:135–42.
41. DeVito EE, Babuscio TA, Nich C, Ball SA, Carroll KM. Gender differences in clinical outcomes for cocaine dependence: randomized clinical trials of behavioral therapy and disulfiram. Drug Alcohol Depend. 2014;145:156–67.
42. Jofre-Bonet M, Sindelar JL, Petrakis IL, Nich C, Frankforter T, Rounsaville BJ, Carroll KM. Cost effectiveness of disulfiram: treating cocaine use in methadone-maintained patients. J Subst Abuse Treat. 2004;26(3):225–32.
43. Haile CN, De La Garza R II, Mahoney JJ III, Nielsen DA, Kosten TR, Newton TF. The impact of disulfiram treatment on the reinforcing effects of cocaine: a randomized clinical trial. PLoS One. 2012;7(11):e47702.
44. Pani PP, Trogu E, Vacca R, Amato L, Vecchi S, Davoli M. Disulfiram for the treatment of cocaine dependence. Cochrane Database Syst Rev 2010;(1);CD007024.
45. Kalayasiri R, Sughondhabirom A, Gueorguieva R, Coric V, Lynch WJ, Morgan PT, Cubells JF, Malison RT. Self-reported paranoia during laboratory binge cocaine self-administration in humans. Pharmacol Biochem Behav. 2006;83(2):249–56.
46. Malcolm R, Olive MF, Lechner W. The safety of disulfiram for the treatment of alcohol and cocaine dependence in randomized clinical trials: guidance for clinical practice. Expert Opin Drug Saf. 2008;7(4):459–72.

47. Roache JD, Kahn R, Newton TF, Wallace CL, Murff WL, De La Garza R II, Rivera O, Anderson A, Mojsiak J, Elkashef A. A double-blind, placebo-controlled assessment of the safety of potential interactions between intravenous cocaine, ethanol, and oral disulfiram. Drug Alcohol Depend. 2011;119(1–2):37–45.
48. Haile CN, During MJ, Jatlow PI, Kosten TR, Kosten TA. Disulfiram facilitates the development and expression of locomotor sensitization to cocaine in rats. Biol Psychiatry. 2003;54(9):915–21.
49. Nagendra SN, Faiman MD, Davis K, Wu JY, Newby X, Schloss JV. Carbamoylation of brain glutamate receptors by a disulfiram metabolite. J Biol Chem. 1997;272(39):24247–51.
50. Kalivas PW, Volkow ND. New medications for drug addiction hiding in glutamatergic neuroplasticity. Mol Psychiatry. 2011;16(10):974–86.
51. Kalivas PW. The glutamate homeostasis hypothesis of addiction. Nat Rev Neurosci. 2009;10(8):561–72.
52. Raylu N, Oei TP. Pathological gambling: a comprehensive review. Clin Psychol Rev. 2002;22(7):1009–61.
53. Hall GW, Carriero NJ, Takushi RY, Montoya ID, Preston KL, Gorelick DA. Pathological gambling among cocaine-dependent outpatients. Am J Psychiatry. 2000;157(7):1127–33.
54. American Psychiatric Association. Diagnostic and statistical manual for the classification of psychiatric disorders – 5th edition (DSM-5). Philadelphia: American Psychiatric Publishing; 2013.
55. Potenza MN. The neurobiology of pathological gambling and drug addiction: an overview and new findings. Philos Trans R Soc Lond B Biol Sci. 2008;363(1507):3181–9.
56. Goudriaan AE, Oosterlaan J, de Beurs E, Van den Brink W. Pathological gambling: a comprehensive review of biobehavioral findings. Neurosci Biobehav Rev. 2004;28(2):123–41.
57. Reuter J, Raedler T, Rose M, Hand I, Gläscher J, Büchel C. Pathological gambling is linked to reduced activation of the mesolimbic reward system. Nat Neurosci. 2005;8(2):147–66.
58. Meyer G, Schwertfeger J, Exton MS, Janssen OE, Knapp W, Stadler MA, Schedlowski M, Krüger TH. Neuroendocrine response to casino gambling in problem gamblers. Psychoneuroendocrinology. 2004;29(10):1272–80.
59. Bergh C, Eklund T, Södersten P, Nordin C. Altered dopamine function in pathological gambling. Psychol Med. 1997;27(2):473–5.
60. Potenza MN, Steinberg MA, Skudlarski P, Fulbright RK, Lacadie CM, Wilber MK, Rounsaville BJ, Gore JC, Wexler BE. Gambling urges in pathological gambling: a functional magnetic resonance imaging study. Arch Gen Psychiatry. 2003;60(8):828–36.
61. Kim SW, Grant JE. An open naltrexone treatment study in pathological gambling disorder. Int Clin Psychopharmacol. 2001;16(5):285–9.
62. Grant JE, Kim SW, Odlaug BL. N-acetyl cysteine, a glutamate-modulating agent, in the treatment of pathological gambling: a pilot study. Biol Psychiatry. 2007;62(6):652–7.
63. Hollander E, Sood E, Pallanti S, Baldini-Rossi N, Baker B. Pharmacological treatments of pathological gambling. J Gambl Stud. 2005;21(1):99–108.
64. Kim SW, Grant JE, Eckert ED, Faris PL, Hartman BK. Pathological gambling and mood disorders: clinical associations and treatment implications. J Affect Disord. 2006;92(1):109–16.
65. Mutschler J, Grosshans M, Bühler M, Diehl A, Kiefer F. Disulfiram in the treatment of pathological gambling? Pharmacopsychiatry. 2009;42(5):110.
66. Mutschler J, Bühler M, Diehl A, Mann K, Kiefer F. Disulfiram, an old drug with new potential in the treatment of pathological gambling? Med Hypotheses. 2010;74(1):209–10.
67. Mutschler J, Bühler M, Grosshans M, Diehl A, Mann K, Kiefer F. Disulfiram, an option for the treatment of pathological gambling? Alcohol Alcohol. 2010;45(2):214–6.

Disulfiram in Comparison and Combination with Other Agents in the Management of Alcohol Dependence

5

5.1 Introduction

Disulfiram is one of the oldest agents used in the pharmacotherapy of alcohol dependence and involves nearly seven decades of clinical experience. The present chapter reviews various studies done where disulfiram has been compared head on to other agents used in the management of alcohol dependence. The chapter also reviews various potential combinations of medications that can be used with disulfiram to supplement and enhance its effect as well as symbiotically enhance the effect of the combination as well.

5.2 Disulfiram in Comparison with Other Agents in Alcohol Dependence

There are very few controlled studies where disulfiram is compared to other agents in the pharmacotherapy of alcohol dependence. Lack of pharma support and funding is a reason for the same. The modest amount of literature available is reviewed in this section.

In a study that compared the efficacy of acamprosate (ACP) and disulfiram (DSF) for preventing alcoholic relapse in routine clinical practice, 100 alcoholic men with family members who would encourage medication compliance and accompany them for follow-up were randomly allocated to 8 months of treatment with DSF or ACP. Weekly group psychotherapy was also available. Alcohol consumption, craving and adverse events were recorded weekly for 3 months and then fortnightly. At the end of the study, 93 patients were still in contact and relapse (the consumption of >5 drinks/40 g of alcohol) occurred at a mean of 123 days with DSF compared to 71 days with ACP. 88% of patients on DSF remained abstinent compared to 46% with ACP. However, patients allocated to ACP had lower craving than those on DSF. This study concluded that DSF is superior to ACP in preventing relapse in alcohol dependence [1].

A. De Sousa, *Disulfiram*, https://doi.org/10.1007/978-981-32-9876-7_5

In another study, to compare the efficacy of naltrexone and disulfiram in preventing an alcoholic relapse in routine clinical practice, 100 alcohol-dependent men, for whom a family member would accompany the patient to follow-up appointments, were randomly allocated to a year of treatment with either naltrexone or disulfiram. Patients, the accompanying family member and the treating psychiatrist were aware of the nature of treatment given. Alcohol consumption, craving and adverse events were recorded weekly for the first 3 months, then fortnightly for the rest of the year, by the treating psychiatrist. At the end of the year, 97 patients were still in contact. Relapse, the consumption of >5 drinks (40 g of ethanol) in a 24 h period, occurred at a mean of 119 days with disulfiram and at 63 days with naltrexone. 86% of the patients remained abstinent throughout the study with disulfiram compared to 44% with naltrexone. Disulfiram was thus regarded as superior to naltrexone in preventing a relapse among alcohol-dependent men with family support [2].

The same authors also compared the efficacy of disulfiram to topiramate for preventing alcoholic relapse in an open study of routine clinical practice in India. One hundred alcohol-dependent men with family members who agreed to encourage medical compliance and to accompany them for follow-up were randomly allocated to 9 months of treatment with disulfiram or topiramate. Weekly psychotherapy was also provided. Supervision and support of the family member were used in the maintenance of compliance among the patients. Alcohol consumption, craving and adverse events were recorded weekly for 3 months and then biweekly. Relapse occurred at a mean of 133 days for disulfiram as compared with 79 days for topiramate. At 9 months, 90% of disulfiram patients as compared with 56% of topiramate patients remained abstinent [3].

In yet another study, in a naturalistic outpatient treatment setting, retrospective data from 2002 to 2007 were analyzed on 353 alcohol-dependent subjects in outpatient treatment, who, according to the patient's and the clinician's mutual decision, received either supervised disulfiram (with thrice-weekly appointments) or acamprosate (once-weekly appointments) following an inpatient alcohol detoxification treatment. Abstinence was assessed by alcohol breathalyzer, patients' self report, urine and serum analyses and overall physicians' rating. Time elapsed before the first alcohol relapse as well as attendance to outpatient treatment and cumulative alcohol abstinence achieved within outpatient treatment was explicitly longer in the disulfiram group. A longer duration of alcohol dependence predicted a favourable treatment outcome in the disulfiram group, while for the acamprosate group the chances for a successful treatment increased with shorter duration of alcohol dependence. This study supports the notion that supervised disulfiram is an important component of alcoholism treatment, and it appears to be more effective than the treatment with acamprosate particularly in patients with a long duration of alcohol dependence [4, 5].

In a study that compared the effects of disulfiram, naltrexone and acamprosate each combined with a brief manual-based cognitive-behavioural intervention a randomized, open-label, multi-centre naturalistic study in two phases was conducted. The first, a 12-week continuously supervised medication, followed by targeted medication up to 52 weeks in addition to a 67-week follow-up period; altogether 119 weeks (2.5 years), in 243 voluntary treatment-seeking alcohol-dependent adult outpatients. They were randomized 1:1:1 to receive supervised naltrexone (50 mg/day), acamprosate (1998 mg/day) and disulfiram (250 mg/day) plus a brief manual-based cognitive-behavioural intervention. The patients were met in the second and sixth weeks, and then after 3, 6 and 12 months. All three study groups showed marked reduction in drinking, from baseline to the end of the study. During the continuous medication phase, treatment with disulfiram was more effective in reducing heavy drinking days and average weekly alcohol consumption, and increasing time to the first drink, as well as the number of abstinent days. Abstinence days were significantly more frequent in the disulfiram group than the other two drugs. Supervised disulfiram appeared superior, especially during the continuous medication period, to both naltrexone and acamprosate.

The studies mentioned above were open-label studies and done in settings that mimicked routine clinical practice. It is also prudent that researchers realize that blinded studies may not possible with disulfiram as the patient knowing that he is on disulfiram and the psychological knowledge and fear of the disulfiram–ethanol reaction are important for disulfiram to work. To the best of our knowledge the studies above are the only studies where there is head on comparisons of disulfiram to other drugs in the management of alcohol dependence.

5.3 Disulfiram Combined with Other Agents in the Alcohol Dependence

This section shall specifically look at studies where disulfiram was combined with other agents in the management of patients with alcohol dependence.

In a double blind, placebo-controlled trial that evaluated the efficacy of disulfiram, naltrexone and their combination in patients with co-occurring cocaine and alcohol dependence, 208 patients were randomized to disulfiram (250 mg/day), naltrexone (100 mg/day), the combination, or placebo for 11 weeks. Patients taking disulfiram (alone or in combination) were most likely to achieve combined abstinence from cocaine and alcohol. Secondary analyses revealed that patients taking the disulfiram–naltrexone combination were most likely to achieve 3 consecutive weeks of abstinence from cocaine and alcohol [6].

In another study 254 patients with an Axis I psychiatric disorder and comorbid alcohol dependence were treated for 12 weeks in an outpatient medication study conducted at three Veterans Administration outpatient clinics. Randomization included assignment to one of four groups: (1) naltrexone alone; (2) placebo alone; (3) (open-label) disulfiram and (blinded) naltrexone or (4) (open-label) disulfiram and (blinded) placebo. There was a high rate of abstinence across groups. Subjects treated with an active medication had significantly more consecutive weeks of abstinence and less craving than those treated with placebo, but there were no significant group differences in other measures of alcohol consumption. There was no advantage of the combination of both medications. The data suggest a modest advantage for the use of disulfiram and naltrexone for this group of dually diagnosed alcohol-dependent individuals [7].

5.4 Combining Disulfiram with Other Drugs—A Clinical Approach

It is often a clinical dilemma whether one must use or multiple medications in the long-term pharmacotherapy of alcohol dependence. This section looks at various drugs that may be combined with disulfiram and the potential advantages and disadvantages of such combinations from a clinical practice perspective.

5.5 Disulfiram and Naltrexone

There are a few advantages of this combination when used in the long-term management of alcohol dependence:

1. Both these drugs act via diverse mechanisms of action with naltrexone being an opioid antagonist with a proven history in reducing euphoria, alcohol intake and reducing the risk of relapse in alcoholic patients [8, 9]. This action is thought to be due to the blockade of mu-opioid receptors. This antagonism prevents the release of endogenous opioids that would, on consumption of alcohol, produce a dopamine surge in the reward centre of the nucleus accumbens of the medulla [10]. Disulfiram on the other hand acts via the inhibition of acetaldehyde dehydrogenase, by blocking the further metabolism of acetaldehyde, which is an intermediate metabolic product of alcohol in the body. The resulting increased acetaldehyde levels in the body lead to the characteristic disulfiram–ethanol reaction (DER), which includes a sense of uneasiness, flushing and a feeling of nausea and vomiting [11]. This diversity in pharmacological action serves to cover different mechanisms in the pathophysiology of alcohol dependence and enhances the effect of both medications when used together.
2. It is also important to note that naltrexone is an anti-craving agent while disulfiram acts as an alcohol deterrent, and thus while one drug may reduce craving the other will prevent the person from drinking in the fear of the disulfiram–ethanol reaction. The dosage in which these drugs are used also play an important role. It is important that naltrexone be prescribed at 50–150 mg/day based on the need and disulfiram be prescribed at 250–500 mg/day [12].
3. One of the disadvantages of this combination is that both disulfiram and naltrexone are hepatotoxic and undergo first-pass metabolism in the liver. One has to be careful when using both these drugs in combination in patients with alcohol dependence that may have compromised liver functions, and thus liver function monitoring must be stringent and mandatory [13, 14].
4. Another point of clinical interest is that both these drugs are also available in depot form in the form of implants. While the efficacy of disulfiram implants in alcohol dependence remains questionable [15], naltrexone has been used with good results as an implant in opioid dependence though its role in alcohol dependence as an implant is under investigation [16].

5.6 Disulfiram and Acamprosate

This is a combination that has similar potential to disulfiram and naltrexone, but some distinct clinical points emerge.

1. The mechanism of action of disulfiram is already known to us as described above, while acamprosate has its own unique mechanism of action via changes in the brain that mimic the effects of NMDA receptor antagonism by some indirect mechanism. This does not exclude changes in GABA transmission, effects on other amino acids in the CNS, or effects on oxidation stress. It has also been demonstrated to have some neuroprotective effects [17, 18].
2. One advantage of acamprosate is that it can be started on the first day during withdrawal itself and can be a part of anti-withdrawal treatment that shall then be carried over to the long-term management of alcohol dependence where disulfiram may be added. Studies have shown that the anti-craving and deterrent combination of these two drugs work well in alcohol dependence [4].
3. It is also worthwhile to realize that disulfiram and acamprosate combined do not have a major effect on the liver and can be used safely. Also, the effect of acamprosate on glutamate opens an unexplored area in alcohol dependence pharmacology and provides neuroprotection from glutamate excitotoxicity that may happen during alcohol withdrawal as well [19]. It is thus a combination that is worth trying in the long-term management of alcohol dependence.

5.7 Disulfiram and Topiramate

Topiramate is one of the newer agents being used in the long-term pharmacotherapy of alcohol dependence with promising results [20]. Some points of clinical interest in this combination are

1. Topiramate may be effective in the management of alcohol dependence as it may decrease dopamine activity in the brain after alcohol intake, partly because of its ability to enhance g-aminobutyric-acid-mediated inhibition through non-benzodiazepine receptors [21]. This is also possible due to its antagonism of glutamate at the 5-amino-3-hydroxy-5-methyl-4-isoxazole propionic acid receptors. Thus, topiramate may counteract the changes that occur at these receptors with chronic alcohol use [22].
2. Topiramate in addition to anti-craving properties has the distinct advantage of being an anticonvulsant. It can thus be started in the anti-withdrawal stage of treatment where it shall perform a triple role of being an anticonvulsant to prevent seizures during alcohol withdrawal, act as a mood stabilizer and prevent mood swings and irritability during alcohol withdrawal while also acting as an anti craving agent. Thus, it can support the patient till disulfiram is added to it in the maintenance phase. Its renal clearance also helps in preventing any effect in form of liver toxicity [23].

3. We have been using this combination in clinical practice in India with a fair amount of success, and topiramate may be cost-effective and a cheaper alternative to naltrexone and acamprosate in many cases. However, when used in alcohol dependence, the patient must be exhorted to drink a lot of water and keep himself hydrated due to the side effect of renal calculi reported in some cases with long-term topiramate use [24].

5.8 Disulfiram and Baclofen

There are no clinical studies of baclofen use with disulfiram in the management of alcohol dependence. This combination is different from the above three in some ways:

1. Neuroanatomically, the reward system in alcohol dependence is constituted of dopaminergic neurons originating in the ventral tegmental area and terminating in the nucleus accumbens and amygdala. These neurons receive GABAergic inputs which have an inhibitory effect on dopaminergic tone that may reduce the reinforcing effects of substances of abuse [25]. Several lines of evidence indicate that alcohol withdrawal hyperexcitability is associated with increased function of the *N*-methyl-D-aspartate subtype of glutamate receptor [26]. The inhibitory action of the GABA B receptor system on neurotransmission also involves the regulation of excitatory amino acid functions; for instance, presynaptic GABA B receptors may inhibit glutamate release, while postsynaptic GABA B receptors may hyperpolarize postsynaptic neurons [27]. This is the mechanism of action of Baclofen in alcohol dependence.
2. Disulfiram could possibly be combined well with Baclofen but we would need data from controlled studies before the same could be concretely ascertained. Baclofen may also be a good alternative in cases where naltrexone or acamprosate are not tolerated or ineffective.

One of the most important factors in combining disulfiram with any agent remains the fact that disulfiram is the only drug that would cause abstinence due to its ability to cause a reaction with alcohol and prevent the patient from drinking. All the other drugs while they reduce craving may still allow the patient to drink or slip while on the drug.

5.9 Conclusion

Disulfiram has been shown in studies to be superior to naltrexone, acamprosate and topiramate in the management of alcohol dependence. The various combinations of drugs that can be used with disulfiram have been elucidated, and clinically and theoretically it does seem that combination of pharmacological agents would work best in the management of alcohol dependence.

References

1. De Sousa A, De Sousa A. An open randomized study comparing disulfiram and acamprosate in the treatment of alcohol dependence. Alcohol Alcohol. 2005;40(6):545–8.
2. De Sousa A, De Sousa A. A one-year pragmatic trial of naltrexone vs disulfiram in the treatment of alcohol dependence. Alcohol Alcohol. 2004;39(6):528–31.
3. De Sousa AA, De Sousa J, Kapoor H. An open randomized trial comparing disulfiram and topiramate in the treatment of alcohol dependence. J Subs Abuse Treat. 2008;34(4):460–3.
4. Diehl A, Ulmer L, Mutschler J, Herre H, Krumm B, Croissant B, Mann K, Kiefer F. Why is disulfiram superior to acamprosate in the routine clinical setting? A retrospective long-term study in 353 alcohol-dependent patients. Alcohol Alcohol. 2010;45(3):271–7.
5. Laaksonen E, Koski-Jännes A, Salaspuro M, Ahtinen H, Alho H. A randomized, multicentre, open-label, comparative trial of disulfiram, naltrexone and acamprosate in the treatment of alcohol dependence. Alcohol Alcohol. 2007;43(1):53–61.
6. Pettinati HM, Kampman KM, Lynch KG, Xie H, Dackis C, Rabinowitz AR, Charles PO. A double blind, placebo-controlled trial that combines disulfiram and naltrexone for treating co-occurring cocaine and alcohol dependence. Addict Behav. 2008;33(5):651–67.
7. Petrakis IL, Poling J, Levinson C, Nich C, Carroll K, Rounsaville B, VA New England VISN I MIRECC Study Group. Naltrexone and disulfiram in patients with alcohol dependence and comorbid psychiatric disorders. Biol Psychiatry. 2005;57(10):1128–37.
8. Kranzler HR, Van Kirk J. Efficacy of naltrexone and acamprosate for alcoholism treatment: a meta-analysis. Alcohol Clin Exp Res. 2001;25(9):1335–41.
9. O'Brien CP, Volpicelli LA, Volpicelli JR. Naltrexone in the treatment of alcoholism: a clinical review. Alcohol. 1996;13(1):35–9.
10. Krystal JH, Cramer JA, Krol WF, Kirk GF, Rosenheck RA. Naltrexone in the treatment of alcohol dependence. N Engl J Med. 2001;345(24):1734–9.
11. Savas MC, Güllü İH. Disulfiram–ethanol test reaction: significance of supervision. Ann Pharmacother. 1997;31(3):374–5.
12. Brewer C, Meyers RJ, Johnsen J. Does disulfiram help to prevent relapse in alcohol abuse? CNS Drugs. 2000;14(5):329–41.
13. Preston KL, Silverman K, Umbricht A, DeJesus A, Montoya ID, Schuster CR. Improvement in naltrexone treatment compliance with contingency management. Drug Alcohol Depend. 1999;54(2):127–35.
14. Poulsen HE, Loft S, Andersen JR, Andersen M. Disulfiram therapy–adverse drug reactions and interactions. Acta Psychiatr Scand. 1992;86(S369):59–66.
15. Wilson A. Disulfiram implantation in alcoholism treatment. A review. J Stud Alcohol. 1975;36(5):555–65.
16. Lobmaier PP, Kunøe N, Gossop M, Waal H. Naltrexone depot formulations for opioid and alcohol dependence: a systematic review. CNS Neurosci Ther. 2011;17(6):629–36.
17. Carmen B, Angeles M, Ana M, María AJ. Efficacy and safety of naltrexone and acamprosate in the treatment of alcohol dependence: a systematic review. Addiction. 2004;99(7):811–28.
18. Mason BJ. Treatment of alcohol-dependent outpatients with acamprosate: a clinical review. J Clin Psychiatry. 2001;62:42–8.
19. Plosker GL. Acamprosate: a review of its use in alcohol dependence. Drugs. 2015;75(11):1255–68.
20. Kenna GA, Lomastro TL, Schiesl A, Leggio L, Swift RM. Review of topiramate: an antiepileptic for the treatment of alcohol dependence. Curr Drug Abuse Rev. 2009;2(2):135–42.
21. De Sousa A. The role of topiramate and other anticonvulsants in the treatment of alcohol dependence: a clinical review. CNS Neurol Disord Drug Targets. 2010;9(1):45–9.
22. Guglielmo R, Martinotti G, Quatrale M, Ioime L, Kadilli I, Di Nicola M, Janiri L. Topiramate in alcohol use disorders: review and update. CNS Drugs. 2015;29(5):383–95.
23. Olmsted CL, Kockler DR. Topiramate for alcohol dependence. Ann Pharmacother. 2008;42(10):1475–80.

24. Lamb EJ, Stevens PE, Nashef L. Topiramate increases biochemical risk of nephrolithiasis. Ann Clin Biochem. 2004;41(2):166–9.
25. Volkow ND, Wang GJ, Fowler JS, Tomasi D, Telang F. Addiction: beyond dopamine reward circuitry. Proc Natl Acad Sci U S A. 2011;108(37):15037–42.
26. Gass JT, Olive MF. Glutamatergic substrates of drug addiction and alcoholism. Biochem Pharmacol. 2008;75(1):218–65.
27. Cruz HG, Ivanova T, Lunn ML, Stoffel M, Slesinger PA, Lüscher C. Bi-directional effects of GABA B receptor agonists on the mesolimbic dopamine system. Nat Neurosci. 2004;7(2):153–9.

Disulfiram and Its Use in Special Populations

6

6.1 Introduction

As noted in previous chapters, disulfiram has been shown to be effective in the management of alcohol dependence and cocaine dependence. This chapter reviews the various studies of disulfiram in special and distinct populations of alcohol-dependent and cocaine-dependent patients with other comorbid disorders. It also reviews the studies of disulfiram in special age groups of patients with these disorders.

6.2 Disulfiram in the Elderly

In an open-label trial, to compare the efficacy of disulfiram and naltrexone for preventing alcoholic relapse in elderly patients in routine clinical practice, 32 elderly alcoholics with proper relatives or caregivers that would encourage medical compliance and would accompany them for follow up were randomly allocated to 6 months of treatment with disulfiram or naltrexone. Weekly group supportive psychotherapy was also provided. The psychiatrist, patient and family member were aware of the treatment prescribed. Alcohol consumption, craving and adverse events were recorded weekly for 2 months and fortnightly thereafter. At the end of the study, 46 patients were still in contact. Relapse occurred at a mean of 91 days with disulfiram compared to 52 days for naltrexone. 81.25% patients on disulfiram remained abstinent compared to 43.75% with naltrexone. Thus, disulfiram was thus found to be superior to naltrexone in preventing relapse in elderly alcoholics with good caregiver support [1]. This is the first exclusive study of disulfiram in a population above the age of 60 years.

Many review papers on the long-term management of alcohol dependence in the elderly are skeptical with regard to the use of disulfiram in the elderly [2–4]. As far as elderly populations are concerned, there are certain precautions, and extreme caution needs to be exercised while prescribing disulfiram. Disulfiram should not be started if there is underlying hepatic dysfunction or if serum glutamic oxaloacetic

A. De Sousa, *Disulfiram*, https://doi.org/10.1007/978-981-32-9876-7_6

transaminase/serum glutamic-pyruvic transaminase are raised twice or thrice above normal. At the time of initiation, one has to ascertain that there is no alcohol use in the preceding at least 12 h [5]. Disulfiram therapy works best if dosing is supervised by a family member to ensure compliance. This may be again a problem with elderly, who may not have adequate social support or whose family members may not have time for supervision or accompany for follow-up. The elderly may often have subtle, age-related cognitive impairments. Further, if there is a risk of ongoing or intermittent alcohol use while on disulfiram, the elderly may experience serious complications, especially if staying alone [6]. Disulfiram is contraindicated in patients with a history of seizures or psychosis, cerebrovascular disease, peripheral neuropathy, etc., which may be otherwise common comorbidities among elderly patients. The use of disulfiram, therefore, may be done only with extreme caution in elderly alcohol users [7].

6.3 Disulfiram Use in Adolescents

In a study to assess the efficacy and safety of long-term disulfiram treatment in alcohol dependence of adolescents, the authors recruited 26 adolescents, aged 16–19 years, with chronic or episodic alcohol dependence. Patients were allocated treatment randomly with disulfiram (200 mg daily) or placebo for 90 days. Patients were assessed on the day treatment started and on days 30 and 90 by interview, self-report, questionnaire and laboratory screening. Time to first treatment failure (relapse or non-attendance) was the primary outcome measure. Thirteen disulfiram-treated and 13 placebo-treated patients completed the treatment phase. At the end of treatment, seven disulfiram-treated and two placebo-treated patients were abstinent continuously. Mean cumulative abstinence duration was significantly greater in the disulfiram group than in the placebo group. It was thus concluded that disulfiram may be an effective and well-tolerated pharmacological adjunct to psychosocial and behavioural treatment programmes for treatment of adolescent alcohol-dependent patients [8].

In another study, 58 adolescents with alcohol dependence having family members that would encourage medical compliance and would accompany them for follow-up were randomly allocated to 6 months of treatment with disulfiram or naltrexone. Weekly psycho-education was also provided. Relapse occurred at a mean of 84 days with disulfiram compared with 51 days for naltrexone. A total of 79.31% patients on disulfiram remained abstinent compared with 51.72% with naltrexone, while patients allocated with naltrexone, however, had less craving than the disulfiram group [9].

However, disulfiram use in adolescents still appears a grey area of clinical practice. Further studies in larger groups and across diverse populations are needed before we reach any firm conclusions regarding its efficacy. Another word of caution with disulfiram use in adolescents is the fact that these groups of patients are rather impulsive and may drink alcohol while on disulfiram increasing the propensity of disulfiram–ethanol reactions.

6.4 Disulfiram in Female Patients and Pregnancy

In a study on disulfiram use in patients with borderline personality disorder where majority of the subjects were female patients, adherence to treatment was 18.44 ± 21.78 months. The first relapse occurred after 1.38 ± 1.41 months. The cumulated time of abstinence was 16.88 ± 20.48 months. The overall tolerability was considered to be high; dizziness and fatigue appeared in all patients at the beginning of the therapy but did not persist. No serious adverse events or ethanol–disulfiram interactions were observed. No suicidal behaviour was reported. Disulfiram was well tolerated in the group [10].

Disulfiram is assumed to be more dangerous in patients with borderline personality disorder since these patients tend to be impulsive, their self-control is reduced and they self-injure and make suicidal threats/attempts more than patients with alcohol dependence without concomitant psychiatric disorders [11]. The fear that patients with borderline personality disorder especially could suffer serious harm by drinking alcohol while taking disulfiram contributes to the common opinion that disulfiram is not suitable for the treatment of alcohol addiction in patients with this personality disorder. However, they are a group who particularly tend to have poor treatment outcomes with higher rates of relapse to alcohol and a greater likelihood for developing alcohol-related problems [12].

In studies of disulfiram in the management of cocaine dependence it has been observed that women, compared with men, had poorer treatment outcomes on multiple measures of cocaine use during treatment and at post-treatment follow-up. These results appear to be primarily accounted for by disulfiram being less effective in women compared with men. There was no evidence of meaningful gender differences in outcome as a function of the behavioural therapies evaluated [13].

In a review that looked at the efficacy of medications in the long-term management of alcohol dependence in female patients, the results showed that the rates of women recruited for studies evaluating the efficacy of disulfiram were too low to establish possible gender differences. The rates of women recruited for studies evaluating the efficacy of drugs like acamprosate and naltrexone were higher and allowed evaluation of data obtained for female patients. Women received medications for treatment of alcohol dependence for which efficacy has been demonstrated in studies in which men were more largely represented [14].

In a review on pharmacotherapy of alcohol dependence in pregnancy, it has been reported that while disulfiram treatment has met with mixed results in controlled studies of nonpregnant adults, patients may not feel capable of abstinence without it and may wish to continue disulfiram for alcohol avoidance during gestation. Because evidence is so scant, it may be prudent to avoid disulfiram during pregnancy [15]. It is postulated that developmental toxicity from high levels of acetaldehyde is possible among pregnant women who drink alcohol and take disulfiram. Non-specific foetal abnormalities have been reported with first trimester exposure, although this effect may be overestimated [16, 17]. The current literature is insufficient to indicate whether congenital abnormalities in disulfiram-exposed fetuses resulted from the drug, alcohol–drug interactions, or other factors [18].

6.5 Disulfiram Use in Patients with Dual Diagnosis

The use of disulfiram for alcohol dependence in the presence of psychiatric illnesses has been debated for two main reasons viz. because the rate of substance use disorders is higher in patients with psychiatric illnesses and especially those with psychotic spectrum disorders like schizophrenia and bipolar disorder [19] and because disulfiram as a side effect can sometimes precipitate symptoms such as depression, mania, psychosis and delirium [20]. Older studies that report that side effects were from the 1970s when disulfiram was being used in large doses, between 1000 and 3000 mg/day [21].

Researchers conducted retrospective comprehensive chart reviews on 33 patients with alcoholism and severe mental illness that included 70% patients of schizophrenia who were maintained on disulfiram. Disulfiram use led to decreases in days hospitalized in patients, and around 64% patients reported remission of alcoholism for at least 1 year during a 3-year follow-up [22]. In another study the authors reported no significant changes in positive, negative or general PANSS scores in subjects with psychotic spectrum disorders who were given disulfiram. They also reported better alcohol-use outcomes for patients with a psychotic spectrum disorder who were on an active medication (disulfiram or naltrexone or combination) compared with placebo but did not report of any advantage of disulfiram or naltrexone or of the combination [23]. This study supports the use of disulfiram for alcohol dependence with comorbid psychotic spectrum disorders, suggesting that these patients benefit more with such treatment methods as they may not be able to benefit fully from the forms of treatments developed for non-comorbid alcohol-dependence patients.

In yet another study [24], it was reported that subjects with depression reported lower craving over time with disulfiram than those on naltrexone. They concluded that disulfiram is safe for patients of alcohol use disorder and comorbid depression. Certain studies speak about reduction in craving with disulfiram therapy, while many others do not support this claim. In a study on alcohol dependence and PTSD, 93 individuals who met DSM- IV-TR criteria for post-traumatic stress disorder (PTSD) reported better alcohol outcomes with active medication (naltrexone, disulfiram, or the combination) wherein overall psychiatric symptoms of PTSD improved [25].

Research suggests that disulfiram can be safely and effectively used with patients who have comorbid diagnoses of Axis I and Axis II disorders (antisocial and borderline personality disorders). Many clinicians fear its use in personality disorders due to increased impulsivity in such patients. A diagnosis of personality disorder did not adversely affect alcohol outcomes and they did not have a poorer response to medications than patients without diagnosis of personality disorders [20]. Many review on the pharmacotherapy of dual diagnosis patients support the use of disulfiram in the long-term management of alcohol dependence in such patients [26, 27]. Clinicians have long recognized that disulfiram is a useful adjunct for the management of alcohol abuse patients because the drug diminishes the risk of impulsive drinking in otherwise well-motivated patients. Careful monitoring and attention to drug interactions may extend this same benefit to schizophrenic patients who abuse alcohol [28]. A recent review on the pharmacotherapy of alcohol dependence in patients with psychotic spectrum disorders also heralds the use of disulfiram in these patients [29]. Similarly a clinical review on the medical management of alcohol dependence and bipolar disorder also supports the use of disulfiram in these patients [30].

6.6 Disulfiram Use in Opioid-Dependent Populations

Disulfiram has been used in some studies where cocaine dependence and alcohol dependence co-exist with opioid use. Sixty-seven cocaine and opioid dependence patients were placed directly in the methadone to ensure compliance for 12 weeks and treated with disulfiram or placebo. Disulfiram was found to be an effective pharmacotherapy for cocaine abuse among methadone-maintained opioid addicts, even in those individuals without comorbid alcohol abuse. Disulfiram inhibits dopamine beta-hydroxylase resulting in an excess of dopamine and decreased synthesis of norepinephrine. Since cocaine is a potent catecholamine re-uptake inhibitor, disulfiram may blunt cocaine craving or alter the high, resulting in a decreased desire to use cocaine [31]. The same results have been found for alcohol and cocaine dependence where the subjects were maintained on buprenorphine [32]. A recent randomized controlled trial has also supported the use of 250 mg disulfiram per day in reducing cocaine use in methadone-stabilized addicts [33].

6.7 Disulfiram in Binge Eating Disorder

There is just one small study on the use of disulfiram in binge eating disorder. 250 mg of disulfiram was administered to 12 patients affected by binge eating disorder for 16 weeks and the number of binge eating episodes per week and the number of participants who reported side effects were evaluated. Nine patients completed the trial, while the other three discontinued prematurely. Disulfiram significantly decreased the mean frequency of binge eating episodes per week and seven participants achieved remission of binge eating. Long-term placebo-controlled studies are warranted to exclude the contribution of a placebo response from these results and to evaluate drugs with similar pharmacological activity but improved tolerability. The effect of disulfiram on dopamine that reduces cocaine craving has been postulated to reduce food craving and hence the potential benefit of disulfiram in binge eating disorder was evaluated [34].

6.8 Positron Emission Tomography Studies with Disulfiram

There is just one early study that looked to neuroimaging with disulfiram use. In a retrospective investigation, the researchers examined the influence of disulfiram administration on the results of PET studies of ICMR glucose and benzodiazepine receptor binding and neuropsychological tests of cognition and executive function in patients with severe chronic alcoholism. [^{18}F]Fluorodeoxyglucose was used to measure lCMRglc in 48 male patients, including 11 receiving and 37 not receiving disulfiram in therapeutic doses. [^{11}C]Flumazenil was used to measure benzodiazepine receptor binding in 17 male patients, including 3 receiving and 14 not receiving disulfiram. All patients studied with FMZ were also examined with fluorodeoxyglucose. PET studies of revealed significantly decreased global values in the patients receiving disulfiram compared with those not receiving disulfiram. PET studies of benzodiazepine receptor binding revealed decreased Flumazenil influx and distribution volume in patients receiving disulfiram. The neuropsychological tests demonstrated no differences between the two groups of subjects. The findings suggest that disulfiram may influence the results of PET studies of glucose metabolism and benzodiazepine receptor binding [35]. No similar studies exist or were repeated after this early paper.

6.9 Conclusion

Disulfiram has been thus used in a wide variety of special populations that consume alcohol with a fair amount of success. Disulfiram is the most common drug that is used for maintenance therapy for alcohol dependence in many Asian settings, as it is cheaper than acamprosate and naltrexone while the reverse is true for Europe and the USA. The cost-effectiveness of disulfiram is another reason where it fits the bill for use in special populations.

References

1. De Sousa A, Jagtap J. An open label trial of naltrexone versus disulfiram in elderly patients with alcohol dependence. J Pak Pychiatr Soc. 2009;6(2):85–9.
2. Menninger JA. Assessment and treatment of alcoholism and substance-related disorders in the elderly. Bull Menn Clin. 2002;66(2):166–83.
3. Dar K. Alcohol use disorders in elderly people: fact or fiction? Adv Psychiatr Treat. 2006;12(3):173–81.
4. Culberson J. Alcohol use in the elderly: beyond the CAGE. Geriatrics. 2006;61(10):23–7.
5. Lal R, Pattanayak RD. Alcohol use in the elderly: issues and considerations. J Geriatr Ment Health. 2017;4(1):4–10.
6. Sarkar S, Parmar A, Chatterjee B. Substance use disorders in the elderly: a review. J Geriatr Ment Health. 2015;2(2):74–82.
7. Ross S. Alcohol use disorders in the elderly. Prim Psychiatry. 2005;12(1):32–40.
8. Niederhofer H, Staffen W. Comparison of disulfiram and placebo in treatment of alcohol dependence of adolescents. Drug Alcohol Rev. 2003;22(3):295–7.
9. De Sousa A, De Sousa A. An open randomized trial comparing disulfiram and naltrexone in adolescents with alcohol dependence. J Subst Use. 2008;13(6):382–8.
10. Mutschler J, Grosshans M, Koopmann A, Hermann D, Diehl A, Mann K, Kiefer F. Supervised disulfiram in relapse prevention in alcohol-dependent patients suffering from comorbid borderline personality disorder—a case series. Alcohol Alcohol. 2010;45(2):146–50.
11. Gunderson JG, Weinberg I, Choi-Kain L. Borderline personality disorder. Focus. 2013;11(2):129–45.

12. Stepp SD, Trull TJ, Sher KJ. Borderline personality features predict alcohol use problems. J Pers Disord. 2005;19(6):711–22.
13. DeVito EE, Babuscio TA, Nich C, Ball SA, Carroll KM. Gender differences in clinical outcomes for cocaine dependence: randomized clinical trials of behavioral therapy and disulfiram. Drug Alcohol Depend. 2014;145:156–67.
14. Agabio R, Campesi I, Pisanu C, Gessa GL, Franconi F. Sex differences in substance use disorders: focus on side effects. Addict Biol. 2016;21(5):1030–42.
15. Rayburn WF, Bogenschutz MP. Pharmacotherapy for pregnant women with addictions. Am J Obstetr Gynecol. 2004;191(6):1885–97.
16. Helmbrecht GD, Hoskins IA. First trimester disulfiram exposure: report of two cases. Am J Perinatol. 1993;10(1):5–7.
17. Reitnauer PJ, Callanan NP, Farber RA, Aylsworth AS. Prenatal exposure to disulfiram implicated in the cause of malformations in discordant monozygotic twins. Teratology. 1997;56(6):358–62.
18. Nora A, Nora J, Blu J. Limb-reduction anomalies in infants born to disulfiram-treated alcoholic mothers. Lancet. 1977;310(8039):664.
19. Drake RE, Essock SM, Shaner A, Carey KB, Minkoff K, Kola L, Lynde D, Osher FC, Clark RE, Rickards L. Implementing dual diagnosis services for clients with severe mental illness. Psychiatr Serv. 2001;52(4):469–76.
20. Larson EW, Olincy A, Rummans TA, Morse RM. Disulfiram treatment of patients with both alcohol dependence and other psychiatric disorders: a review. Alcohol Clin Exp Res. 1992;16(1):125–30.
21. Rossiter SK. Psychosis with disulfiram prescribed under probation order. BMJ. 1992;305(6856):763–4.
22. Mueser KT, Noordsy DL, Fox L, Wolfe R. Disulfiram treatment for alcoholism in severe mental illness. Am J Addict. 2003;12(3):242–52.
23. Petrakis IL, Poling J, Levinson C, Nich C, Carroll K, Rounsaville B, VA New England VISN I MIRECC Study Group. Naltrexone and disulfiram in patients with alcohol dependence and comorbid psychiatric disorders. Biol Psychiatry. 2005;57(10):1128–37.
24. Petrakis I, Ralevski E, Nich C, Levinson C, Carroll K, Poling J, Rounsaville B, VA VISN I MIRECC Study Group. Naltrexone and disulfiram in patients with alcohol dependence and current depression. J Clin Psychopharmacol. 2007;27(2):160–5.
25. Petrakis IL, Poling J, Levinson C, Nich C, Carroll K, Ralevski E, Rounsaville B. Naltrexone and disulfiram in patients with alcohol dependence and comorbid post-traumatic stress disorder. Biol Psychiatry. 2006;60(7):777–83.
26. Kranzler HR, Rosenthal RN. Dual diagnosis: alcoholism and co-morbid psychiatric disorders. Am J Addict. 2003;12:26–40.
27. Gual A. Dual diagnosis in Spain. Drug Alcohol Rev. 2007;26(1):65–71.
28. Kingsbury SJ, Salzman C. Disulfiram in the treatment of alcoholic patients with schizophrenia. Psychiatr Serv. 1990;41(2):133–4.
29. Petrakis IL, Nich C, Ralevski E. Psychotic spectrum disorders and alcohol abuse: a review of pharmacotherapeutic strategies and a report on the effectiveness of naltrexone and disulfiram. Schizophr Bull. 2006;32(4):644–54.
30. Farren CK, Hill KP, Weiss RD. Bipolar disorder and alcohol use disorder: a review. Curr Psychiatry Rep. 2012;14(6):659–66.
31. Petrakis IL, Carroll KM, Nich C, Gordon LT, McCance-Katz EF, Frankforter T, Rounsaville BJ. Disulfiram treatment for cocaine dependence in methadone-maintained opioid addicts. Addiction. 2000;95(2):219–28.
32. George TP, Chawarski MC, Pakes J, Carroll KM, Kosten TR, Schottenfeld RS. Disulfiram versus placebo for cocaine dependence in buprenorphine-maintained subjects: a preliminary trial. Biol Psychiatry. 2000;47(12):1080–6.
33. Oliveto A, Poling J, Mancino MJ, Feldman Z, Cubells JF, Pruzinsky R, Gonsai K, Cargile C, Sofuoglu M, Chopra MP, Gonzalez-Haddad G. Randomized, double blind, placebo-controlled

trial of disulfiram for the treatment of cocaine dependence in methadone-stabilized patients. Drug Alcohol Depend. 2011;113(2–3):184–91.
34. Farci AM, Piras S, Murgia M, Chessa A, Restivo A, Gessa GL, Agabio R. Disulfiram for binge eating disorder: an open trial. Eat Behav. 2015;16:84–7.
35. Gilman S, Adams KM, Johnson-Greene D, Koeppe RA, Junck L, Kluin KJ, Martorello S, Heumann M, Hill E. Effects of disulfiram on positron emission tomography and neuropsychological studies in severe chronic alcoholism. Alcohol Clin Exp Res. 1996;20(8):1456–61.

7 Disulfiram: Side Effects and Toxicity

7.1 Introduction

Disulfiram has been used widely in the management of alcohol and/or cocaine dependence. There have been many common and uncommon side effects reported with the drug. The current chapter clinically reviews side effects like liver toxicity, neuropathy, psychosis and catatonia that may be seen with disulfiram. Some facets of the disulfiram–ethanol reaction are also discussed and guidelines for the management of the reaction and side effects are suggested.

7.2 Liver Toxicity

Disulfiram undergoes metabolism through the liver and thus one has to be cautious when using the drug in patients with alcohol dependence that may have already deranged liver function. There have been many case reports of disulfiram-induced hepatitis; the risk of mortality with this hepatitis is very low and has been estimated to be 1 case in 30,000 treated patients per year [1]. Researchers in a review have written against the decision to refrain from prescribing disulfiram for the fear of causing hepatotoxicity [2]. It is known that disulfiram-induced liver toxicity is not dose-dependent and can even occur at low doses and is seen between 16–120 days after the start of medication and usually manifests within 60 days of treatment [3]. As a routine, baseline liver function tests must be carried out prior to starting disulfiram and repeat testing at every 2 weeks for the first month, monthly for 3 months and every 3 months thereafter [4]. It is also important that time is not lost during the initial days because of liver function, as the patient's motivation to leave alcohol and start disulfiram may be high. Thus sometimes, one may clinically evaluate liver dysfunction (signs of liver damage in alcohol dependence) and check hepatomegaly clinically before starting the patient on disulfiram after proper patient psychoeducation [5].

A. De Sousa, *Disulfiram*, https://doi.org/10.1007/978-981-32-9876-7_7

There have been over 30–35 case reports of disulfiram-induced hepatitis in literature. Female patients have been more prone to disulfiram-induced liver damage and one wonders whether women are more susceptible to this toxicity than are men. Predominant symptoms of disulfiram-induced liver damage include fatigue, malaise, anorexia, nausea and jaundice, with accompanying fever, abdominal pain, rash or pruritus in some cases. There have also been marked elevations of serum AST and/or serum ALT and serum bilirubin. The elevated bilirubin comes back to normal within 2 weeks of stopping disulfiram, while liver enzymes may take 3–4 months to normalize [6]. Recurrence of liver enzyme elevation has been reported on restarting disulfiram in patients. It has been suggested that the mechanism of hepatotoxicity produced by disulfiram is an allergic or hypersensitivity reaction [7]. This occurs in a small number of patients and there is no relationship between dosage and the degree of symptoms [8]. Biopsy from disulfiram-induced liver injury has revealed both hepatocellular and canalicular involvement with enlarged portal tracts, slight fibrosis and infiltrates, including eosinophils. Because alcohol can produce liver toxicity with a similar clinical presentation, it sometimes is difficult to determine the exact causative agent if the patient continues to drink despite disulfiram [9]. Treatment of disulfiram-induced liver injury includes immediate withdrawal of the drug and general supportive measures. Anti-histamines may be started, and generally the prognosis is good if the liver involvement is discovered in time [10].

7.3 Neuropathy

Polyneuropathy and toxic optic neuropathy have both been reported with disulfiram, and this symptom reverses completely with the stoppage or withdrawal of the drug. Adverse reactions in the peripheral nervous system include peripheral neuritis and peripheral neuropathy. This reaction is dose-dependent and related to an accumulation of carbon disulfide, which is a by-product of the metabolism of disulfiram in the liver [11]. Disulfiram neuropathy has been histologically viewed as a distal axonopathy related to the dying-back effect of axonal degeneration [12, 13]. The adverse reaction of peripheral neuropathy is uncommon with disulfiram use. Clinically, disulfiram-induced neuropathy and alcoholic neuropathy can be difficult to distinguish. Some observations that can help include a history of onset that occurs in a matter of weeks in disulfiram neuropathy as opposed to an insidious course over months in alcoholic neuropathy. The progression of the disorder is faster in disulfiram neuropathy [14]. Every year, about 1 in 15,000 patients taking disulfiram will develop neuropathy [15]. Many patients may have sub-clinical alcoholic neuropathy that may be exacerbated and occurs with combined disulfiram-induced neuropathy. The malnutrition seen in patients with alcohol dependence like vitamin B group deficiencies, which is a common comorbidity in alcohol dependence must be excluded via laboratory screening [16]. Some studies also propose decrements in nerve ethanolamine, serine, inositol and glycerophospholipids are a cause of neuropathy [17]. The neuropathy is usually polyneuritis with sensory, motor, or both deficits and in rare cases quadriplegia with complete recovery in 1–5 months after stopping disulfiram. Complete recovery of disulfiram-induced severe optic neuritis usually occurs within 2 months of its discontinuation. To the best of our knowledge, irreversible optic neuropathy/neuritis has not been reported in literature [18].

7.4 Psychosis

Psychoses, including Capgras delusions are known to occur either during or after the use of disulfiram [19]. It is known that disulfiram-induced psychosis can occur in patients without any previous history of psychosis, but it is more common if there is pre-existing vulnerability in the individual such as a positive family history of psychosis or if higher doses of disulfiram are used [20]. Literature reveals that psychosis caused by disulfiram is more common in the Indian settings than in Western ones. The reasons for the same are unknown though it could be cultural differences in neurobiology and genetic polymorphisms in liver metabolism pathways that need to be investigated [21].

Disulfiram's major metabolite diethyldithiocarbamate is an inhibitor of dopamine beta hydroxylase (DBH), an enzyme that catalyzes the metabolism of dopamine to norepinephrine. By inhibiting this metabolic pathway, disulfiram results in an increase of dopamine concentrations in mesolimbic system resulting in psychosis [22]. Risk factors for development of disulfiram-related psychotic symptoms include past history of psychosis or schizophrenia, family history of psychosis or schizophrenia, a rapid increase in dosage, greater than recommended total dosage, old age, past history of drug-induced psychosis or disulfiram-induced psychosis, impaired liver function and concurrent dopaminergic medications or psychostimulant abuse [23]. Alcohol dependence is shown to occur more frequently in the first-degree relatives of patients with bipolar disorder, psychosis and schizophrenia. Thus, alcohol-dependent patients with a family history of psychosis are likely to be more vulnerable to precipitants of psychosis like disulfiram [24].

7.5 Catatonia

The association between catatonia and disulfiram was observed first by Rolf Gjessing in 1965. Therapeutic doses of disulfiram can induce catatonia with or without accompanying psychosis or mood disorder. There are few anecdotal case reports of disulfiram-induced catatonic syndrome, all of which were characterized by stupor, mutism and a few other psychomotor phenomena [25]. The risk of catatonia is increased when excessive amounts of the drug are ingested, the patient is already suffering from a major psychiatric illness or the patient has anatomical brain lesions [26]. In one study, the authors reported three cases of disulfiram-induced Parkinsonism and frontal lobe like syndrome. Symptoms developed either after an acute high dose of disulfiram or after several days to weeks of disulfiram treatment and persisted over several years in two patients [27]. They also found bilateral lesions of the lentiform nuclei on neuroimaging suggesting that basal ganglia are the major targets of disulfiram neurotoxicity. The mechanisms of the lesions of basal ganglia may involve carbon disulfide toxicity [28]. Catatonia has also been reported as variant of disulfiram-induced encephalopathy [29]. In most cases it has been reversible after symptomatic management and stoppage of the drug and is a result of dopamine excess caused by dopamine metabolism inhibition by disulfiram.

7.6 Other Side Effects

Few case reports on disulfiram-induced reversible hypertension have shown that the condition has resolved on withdrawal of the drug. The central nervous system inhibition of dopamine beta hydroxylase leads to reduction in norepinephrine synthesis that interferes with central alpha adrenergic receptor activity leading to the hypertension [30, 31].

A recent study has also reported sexual dysfunction in 6.7–10% of patients receiving disulfiram. Arousal deficits, erectile dysfunction and orgasmic difficulties have been reported. It is difficult to ascertain whether these dysfunctions were purely disulfiram induced and/or partly related to alcohol use [32, 33].

There is one case report of myoclonic seizures caused by disulfiram. The mechanism of seizures associated with disulfiram is not known. The most important toxic metabolites are disulfiram are diethyldithiocarbamate (DDC) and its metabolite, carbon disulfide. DDC chelates copper, thus impairing the activity of dopamine beta hydroxylase and the neuronal toxicity caused by carbon disulfide has been implicated in the causation of seizures [34].

Few cases of overdoses with disulfiram have been reported. There is a case of disulfiram-induced acute encephalopathy caused by its metabolites. The diagnosis of disulfiram poisoning is difficult as it is rapidly cleared from the circulation; its metabolites can be measured only by highly specialized laboratory techniques, which are not readily available [35]. There is no specific antidote for disulfiram toxicity. The exact mechanism of disulfiram-mediated encephalopathy is not known. However, disulfiram metabolites diethyldithiocarbamate and carbon disulfide have been shown to inhibit the activity of the enzyme dopamine-beta-hydroxylase leading to the accumulation of dopamine, producing a relative deficiency of adrenaline and noradrenaline in the area of the basal ganglia. Dopamine-mediated cellular injury may be related to its ability to induce excitotoxic effects of glutamate, calcium-mediated cell death, and impairs the cellular ability to eliminate free oxygen radicals that have been implicated in the genesis of encephalopathy [36].

Prolonged coma with disulfiram overdose has been noted. The ability of its metabolites to chelate copper may provide another mechanism for the neurotoxicity seen with both acute intoxication and chronic use of disulfiram. Lesions of the basal ganglia have been described in patients with extrapyramidal symptoms after therapy with disulfiram [37]. Abnormal accumulation of copper in the central nervous system leading to oxidative stress and neuronal cell death is responsible for this [38]. Carbon disulfide has also been suggested to be responsible for the lesions of basal ganglia by inducing a severe microangiopathy [39]. A few case reports mention a pronounced flaccid quadriparesis after acute disulfiram intoxication have also been reported [40]. Breath may have an odor of garlic or sulphur following therapeutic use and is the result of the presence of acetone and carbon disulfide which are mainly excreted through the lungs. This finding is the basis of a breath test to assess compliance with disulfiram therapy [41].

7.7 Disulfiram–Ethanol Reactions

Symptoms of the disulfiram–ethanol reaction occur mainly due to the histamine like effects of the accumulated acetaldehyde [42]. The symptoms begin within 5–15 min after ingestion of ethanol in patients who have taken disulfiram 3–123 h earlier [43]. The symptoms include flushing, sweating, nausea, vomiting, palpitations, dyspnea and hyperventilation, tremors, confusion, restlessness, drowsiness and hypotension. All these symptoms are usually self-limiting except for hypotension that can sometimes be severe and life-threatening [44]. There have been reports of rare cases of acute myocardial infarction [45] and ischemic stroke [46] due to the disulfiram–ethanol reaction. An interesting observation has also been made by authors [47] to improve detection of any unheralded consumption of alcohol in small quantity by the patient maintained on disulfiram. Monitoring of urinary ethylglucuronide (ETG) improved detection of abstinence in such patients thereby also improving safety by preventing chronic acetaldehyde exposure which has carcinogenic, neurotoxic, and cardiotoxic properties [47]. The management of the disulfiram–ethanol reaction includes supportive measures such as Trendelenberg position, oxygen, intravenous fluids and norepinephrine that is considered as the pressor agent of choice [48]. 4-Methylpyrazole is an alcohol dehydrogenase inhibitor that inhibits the accumulation of acetaldehyde in case of disulfiram–alcohol reaction and leads to improvement in symptoms such as facial flushing and tachycardia [49]. Fomepizole, a first line antidote for methanol poisoning is also a potent inhibitor of alcohol dehydrogenase and has been reported of use in the management of disulfiram–ethanol reactions [50].

Many medications have been implicated in the genesis of disulfiram-like reactions. The activity of aldehyde dehydrogenase 2 is inhibited by disulfiram, chloramphenicol and furazolidone, but not by metronidazole or quinacrine [51]. In addition, although well known for metronidazole, quinacrine also did not increase blood acetaldehyde after ethanol administration. Except disulfiram, all the above drugs increased the levels of brain serotonin. Metronidazole and quinacrine do not produce a typical disulfiram-like reaction, because they do not inhibit hepatic aldehyde dehydrogenase nor increase blood acetaldehyde [52].

Rare complications of the disulfiram–ethanol reaction include myocardial infarction [53], hypertension, bronchospasm and methemoglobinemia [54, 55]. Esophageal rupture [56] and intracranial hemorrhage secondary to profound vomiting may occur [57]. Deaths due to the disulfiram–ethanol reaction have also been reported with disulfiram, cefuroxime and metronidazole [58, 59].

7.8 Disulfiram-Induced Skin Reactions

Some minor skin reactions with disulfiram as a drug have been reported. Maculopapular rashes, flushing and skin eruptions have been reported as a part of the disulfiram–ethanol reaction. Some patients also show an allergic hypersensitivity to the drug and may manifest with minor skin reactions. To the best of our knowledge there are no fatal skin reactions reported with disulfiram [60, 61]. Urticaria and angioedema have been reported with disulfiram in patients that are allergic to nickel where even episodes of cutaneous vasculitis have been reported [62].

7.9 Mortality with Disulfiram

In a study where 1131 adverse event reports related to disulfiram were compiled from national centers around the world, it has been reported that 14 deaths have been reported from disulfiram–ethanol reactions. This is less when we look at the number of patients where the drug has been used. The rate of death from these reactions have been estimated at 1 death per 25,000 patients treated per year [63].

7.10 Conclusion

This chapter has looked at various side effects of disulfiram and toxicity from overdoses. The common side effects like liver toxicity, neuropathy and psychosis along with rare and uncommon side effects are discussed. It is prudent that clinicians should not be afraid to use disulfiram in the light of these side effects, as the failure to use disulfiram has far reaching consequences compared to the side effects. This chapter serves as a guideline to describe the various side effects of disulfiram and exhorts clinicians to use the drug more despite the side effects that may be present.

References

1. Chick J. Safety issues concerning the use of disulfiram in treating alcohol dependence. Drug Saf. 1999;20(5):427–35.
2. Wright C, Vafier JA, Lake CR. Disulfiram-induced fulminating hepatitis: guidelines for liver-panel monitoring. J Clin Psychiatry. 1988;49(11):430–4.
3. Kalra G, De Sousa A, Shrivastava A. Disulfiram in the management of alcohol dependence: a comprehensive clinical review. Open J Psychiatry. 2014;4(1):43.
4. Björnsson E, Nordlinder H, Olsson R. Clinical characteristics and prognostic markers in disulfiram-induced liver injury. J Hepatol. 2006;44(4):791–7.
5. Iber FL, Lee K, Lacoursiere R, Fuller R. Liver toxicity encountered in the Veterans Administration trial of disulfiram in alcoholics. Alcohol Clin Exp Res. 1987;11(3):301–4.
6. Forns X, Caballería J, Bruguera M, Salmerón JM, Vilella A, Mas A, Parés A, Rodés J. Disulfiram-induced hepatitis. Report of four cases and review of the literature. J Hepatol. 1994;21(5):853–7.
7. Petersen EN. The pharmacology and toxicology of disulfiram and its metabolites. Acta Psychiatr Scand. 1992;86(S369):7–13.

8. Eisen HJ, Ginsberg AL. Disulfiram hepatotoxicity. Ann Intern Med. 1975;83(5):673–5.
9. Vazquez JJ, Pardo-Mindan J. Liver cell injury (bodies similar to Lafora's) in alcoholics treated with disulfiram (Antabuse). Histopathology. 1979;3(5):377–84.
10. Verge C, Lucena MI, López-Torres E, Puche-García MJ, Fraga E, Romero-Gomez M, Andrade RJ. Adverse hepatic reactions associated with calcium carbimide and disulfiram therapy: is there still a role for these drugs. World J Gastroenterol. 2006;12(31):5078–83.
11. Filosto M, Tentorio M, Broglio L, Buzio S, Lazzarini C, Pasolini MP, Cotelli MS, Scarpelli M, Mancuso M, Choub A, Padovani A. Disulfiram neuropathy: two cases of distal axonopathy. Clin Toxicol. 2008;46(4):314–6.
12. Mohapatra S, Sahoo MR, Rath N. Disulfiram-induced neuropathy: a case report. Gen Hosp Psychiatry. 2015;37(1):97–9.
13. Tran AT, Rison RA, Beydoun SR. Disulfiram neuropathy: two case reports. J Med Case Rep. 2016;10(1):72.
14. Orakzai A, Guerin M, Beatty S. Disulfiram-induced transient optic and peripheral neuropathy: a case report. Ir J Med Sci. 2007;176(4):319–21.
15. Kulkarni RR, Pradeep AV, Bairy BK. Disulfiram-induced combined irreversible anterior ischemic optic neuropathy and reversible peripheral neuropathy: a prospective case report and review of the literature. J Neuropsychiatr Clin Neurosci. 2013;25(4):339–42.
16. Santos T, Campos AM, Morais H. Sensory-motor axonal polyneuropathy involving cranial nerves: an uncommon manifestation of disulfiram toxicity. Clin Neurol Neurosurg. 2017;152:12–5.
17. Barth KS, Malcolm RJ. Disulfiram: an old therapeutic with new applications. CNS Neurol Disord Drug Targets. 2010;9(1):5–12.
18. De JS, Caparros-Lefebvre D, Nkenjuo JB, Hurtevent JF, Petit H. Acute and reversible myoclonic encephalopathy, extrapyramidal syndrome, polyneuropathy caused by chronic disulfiram poisoning. Rev Neurol. 1995;151(11):667–9.
19. Mohapatra S, Rath NR. Disulfiram induced psychosis. Clin Psychopharmacol Neurosci. 2017;15(1):68–70.
20. Melo RC, Lopes R, Alves JC. A case of psychosis in disulfiram treatment for alcoholism. Case Rep Psychiatry. 2014;2014:561092.
21. Sherif PA, Murthy KK. Psychosis and enuresis during disulfiram therapy. Indian J Psychiatry. 2006;48(1):62–5.
22. Luykx JJ, Vis R, Tijdink JK, Dirckx M, Van Hecke J, Vinkers CH. Psychotic symptoms after combined metronidazole-disulfiram use. J Clin Psychopharmacol. 2013;33(1):136–7.
23. Malcolm R, Olive MF, Lechner W. The safety of disulfiram for the treatment of alcohol and cocaine dependence in randomized clinical trials: guidance for clinical practice. Expert Opin Drug Saf. 2008;7(4):459–72.
24. Spiegel DR, McCroskey A, Puaa K, Meeker G, Hartman L, Hudson J, Hung YC. A case of disulfiram-induced psychosis in a previously asymptomatic patient maintained on mixed amphetamine salts: a review of the literature and possible pathophysiological explanations. Clin Neuropharmacol. 2016;39(5):272–5.
25. Goswami HK, Bhuyan D, Talukdar B. Catatonia induced by disulfiram. Open J Psychiatry Allied Sci. 2015;6(2):143–5.
26. Balaban OD, Atagun MI, Alpkan LR. A case of catatonia induced by disulfiram. J Psychiatr Neurol Sci. 2010;23:215–8.
27. Laplane D, Attal N, Sauron B, de Billy A, Dubois B. Lesions of basal ganglia due to disulfiram neurotoxicity. J Neurol Neurosurg Psychiatry. 1992;55:925–9.
28. Fuller RK, Gordis E. Does disulfiram have a role in alcoholism treatment today? Addiction. 2004;99(1):21–4.
29. Nayak V, Chogtu B, Virupaksha D, Bhandary PV. Disulfiram induced catatonia. Case Study Case Rep. 2011;1:6–8.
30. Kulkarni RR, Bairy BK. Disulfiram induced reversible hypertension: a prospective case study and brief review. Indian J Psychol Med. 2010;35(4):217–9.

31. Rogers WK, Benowitz NL, Wilson KM, Abbott JA. Effect of disulfiram on adrenergic function. Clin Pharmacol Ther. 1979;25(4):469–75.
32. Grover S, Mattoo SK, Pendharkar S, Kandappan V. Sexual dysfunction in patients with alcohol and opioid dependence. Indian J Psychol Med. 2014;36(4):355–65.
33. Jensen SB. Sexual function and dysfunction in younger married alcoholics: a comparative study. Acta Psychiatr Scand. 1984;69(6):543–9.
34. Daniel DG, Swallows A, Wolff F. Capgras delusion and seizures in association with therapeutic dosages of disulfiram. South Med J. 1987;80(12):1577–9.
35. Tartara E, Fanucchi S, D'Errico I, Farina LM, Casoni F, Sinforiani E, Micieli G, Costa A. A case of Wernicke encephalopathy combined with disulfiram intoxication. Cogn Behav Neurol. 2013;26(2):93–8.
36. Borrett D, Ashby P, Bilbao J, Carlen P. Reversible, late-onset disulfiram-induced neuropathy and encephalopathy. Ann Neurol. 1985;17(4):396–9.
37. Krauss JK, Mohadjer M, Wakhloo AK, Mundinger F. Dystonia and akinesia due to pallidoputaminal lesions after disulfiram intoxication. Mov Disord. 1991;6(2):166–70.
38. Rae C, Tesson M, Babich JW, Boyd M, Sorensen A, Mairs RJ. The role of copper in disulfiram-induced toxicity and radiosensitization of cancer cells. J Nucl Med. 2013;54(6):953–60.
39. Haley TJ. Disulfiram (tetraethylthioperoxydicarbonic diamide): a reappraisal of its toxicity and therapeutic application. Drug Metab Rev. 1979;9(2):319–35.
40. Zorzon M, Masè G, Biasutti E, Vitrani B, Cazzato G. Acute encephalopathy and polyneuropathy after disulfiram intoxication. Alcohol Alcohol. 1995;30(5):629–31.
41. Fletcher K, Stone E, Mohamad MW, Faulder GC, Faulder RM, Jones K, Morgan D, Wegerdt J, Kelly M, Chick J. A breath test to assess compliance with disulfiram. Addiction. 2006;101(12):1705–10.
42. Kitson TM. The disulfiram-ethanol reaction: a review. J Stud Alcohol. 1977;38(1):96–113.
43. Fuller RK, Branchey L, Brightwell DR, Derman RM, Emrick CD, Iber FL, James KE, Lacoursiere RB, Lee KK, Lowenstam I, Maany I. Disulfiram treatment of alcoholism: a Veterans Administration cooperative study. JAMA. 1986;256(11):1449–55.
44. Williams CS, Woodcock KR. Do ethanol and metronidazole interact to produce a disulfiram-like reaction? Ann Pharmacother. 2000;34(2):255–7.
45. Karamanakos PN, Pappas P, Boumba VA, Thomas C, Malamas M, Vougiouklakis T, Marselos M. Pharmaceutical agents known to produce disulfiram-like reaction: effects on hepatic ethanol metabolism and brain monoamines. Int J Toxicol. 2007;26(5):423–32.
46. Suh JJ, Pettinati HM, Kampman KM, O'Brien CP. The status of disulfiram: a half of a century later. J Clin Psychopharmacol. 2006;26(3):290–302.
47. Mutschler J, Grosshans M, Koopmann A, Mann K, Kiefer F, Hermann D. Urinary ethylglucuronide assessment in patients treated with disulfiram: a tool to improve verification of abstention and safety. Clin Neuropharmacol. 2010;33(6):285–7.
48. Bourcier S, Mongardon N, Daviaud F, Moachon L, Arnould MA, Perruche F, Pène F, Cariou A. Disulfiram ethanol reaction mimicking anaphylactic, cardiogenic, and septic shock. Am J Emerg Med. 2013;31(1):270–1.
49. Lindros KO, Stowell A, Pikkarainen P, Salaspuro M. The disulfiram (Antabuse)-alcohol reaction in male alcoholics: its efficient management by 4-methylpyrazole. Alcohol Clin Exp Res. 1981;5(4):528–30.
50. Sande M, Thompson D, Monte AA. Fomepizole for severe disulfiram-ethanol reactions. Am J Emerg Med. 2012;30(1):262–e3.
51. Ren S, Cao Y, Zhang X, Jiao S, Qian S, Liu P. Cephalosporin induced disulfiram-like reaction: a retrospective review of 78 cases. Int Surg. 2014;99(2):142–6.
52. O'Shea B. Disulfiram revisited. Hosp Med. 2000;61(12):849–51.
53. Altun G, Altun A, Erdogan O. Acute myocardial infarction due to disulfiram (antabus)–alcohol interaction. Cardiovasc Drugs Ther. 2006;20(5):391–2.
54. Rothrock JF, Johnson PC, Rothrock SM, Merkley R. Fulminant polyneuritis after overdose of disulfiram and ethanol. Neurology. 1984;34(3):357–60.

55. Stransky G, Lambing MK, Simmons GT, Robinson A. Methemoglobinemia in a fatal case of disulfiram-ethanol reaction. J Anal Toxicol. 1997;21(2):178–9.
56. Fernandez D. Another esophageal rupture after alcohol and disulfiram. N Engl J Med. 1972;286(11):610–2.
57. Banys P. The clinical use of disulfiram (Antabuse®): a review. J Psychoactive Drugs. 1988;20(3):243–61.
58. Poulsen HE, Loft S, Andersen JR, Andersen M. Disulfiram therapy–adverse drug reactions and interactions. Acta Psychiatr Scand. 1992;86(S369):59–66.
59. Brewer C. Recent developments in disulfiram treatment. Alcohol Alcohol. 1993;28(4):383–95.
60. Haddock NF, Wilkin JK. Cutaneous reactions to lower aliphatic alcohols before and during disulfiram therapy. Arch Dermatol. 1982;118(3):157–9.
61. Palatty PL, Saldanha E. Status of disulfiram in present day alcoholic deaddiction therapy. Indian J Psychiatry. 2011;53(1):25–9.
62. Brewer C, Hardt F. Preventing disulfiram hepatitis in alcohol abusers: inappropriate guidelines and the significance of nickel allergy. Addict Biol. 1999;4(3):303–8.
63. Brewer C, Streel E, Skinner M. Supervised disulfiram's superior effectiveness in alcoholism treatment: ethical, methodological, and psychological aspects. Alcohol Alcohol. 2017;1:1–7.

Disulfiram: Clinical Pearls, Ethics and Future Needs

8

8.1 Introduction

Disulfiram has been used for over 60 years in the long-term management of alcohol dependence [1]. Disulfiram effectively deters alcohol consumption by inhibiting the enzyme aldehyde dehydrogenase (ALDH). Alcohol dehydrogenase (ADH) converts ethanol to acetaldehyde, which is then converted by ALDH to acetic acid and carbon dioxide. ALDH inhibition causes a marked rise in blood acetaldehyde levels with unpleasant effects such as flushing, nausea, vomiting and headache that constitute the disulfiram–ethanol reaction (DER) [2]. Thus, disulfiram effectively prevents a patient who is on the drug from drinking further unlike other drugs in the long-term management that primarily have an anti-craving action alone.

8.2 Clinical Pearls on Disulfiram

This section is a guide for the busy clinician on the basic tenets when it comes to disulfiram in the management of alcohol/cocaine dependence.

1. Disulfiram is a drug that has been used in thousands of patients over the years and its efficacy and safety has been well established. There are a large number of clinical studies and open-label trials that have demonstrated the efficacy of disulfiram in the long-term management of alcohol dependence and cocaine dependence [3, 4].
2. A very important facet apart from the disulfiram–ethanol reaction and the deterrent action of the drug is the fact that the patient must know he is on disulfiram. Knowledge and proper psychoeducation on the part of the doctor plays a key role in the patient developing a know-how of the disulfiram–ethanol reaction and the fear of the reaction also psychologically deters the patient from drinking. This is also one of the reasons that patients must be aware and hence

A. De Sousa, *Disulfiram*, https://doi.org/10.1007/978-981-32-9876-7_8

randomized double-blind placebo controlled trials are not possible with disulfiram where patient knowing that he is on the medication is vital to its action [5].
3. Non-compliance has been cited as one of the main reasons that patients give up on disulfiram as a treatment. Patients may be deterred by the planned or unplanned experience of a disulfiram–ethanol reaction or more usually by learning about it from the prescribing physician, the internet or other alcoholics. Disulfiram is often described as *'aversive'* and the treatment is often confused with aversion therapy, but deterrence and aversion are very different psychological processes. In particular, while aversion therapy involves repeated exposure to an unpleasant stimulus, most patients never experience the disulfiram–ethanol reaction and do not need to [6].
4. The evidence base for disulfiram has now been subjected to three meta-analyses. In one where ten studies were evaluated, the authors concluded that supervised disulfiram, typically combined with appropriate psychosocial interventions, is effective and probably more effective than the main current alternative medications naltrexone, acamprosate and topiramate [7]. Another large meta-analysis of treatments for substance abuse came to similar conclusions [8]. The most recent meta-analysis in 2014 with 23 studies had no doubt as to disulfiram efficacy for maintaining abstinence or preventing relapse [9].
5. The ability of supervised disulfiram therapy to facilitate abstinence every day, despite powerful real-life temptations, has certain proximal advantages over more distal methods such as Alcoholic Anonymous meetings and regular psychotherapy sessions and relapse prevention training. With exposure to high-risk situations, patients learn how to deal with them when on disulfiram therapy. Disulfiram can be safely combined with any psychosocial intervention like cognitive behaviour therapy, family therapy and other forms of individual psychotherapy [10].
6. Disulfiram is a deterrent and it deters drinking in just the same way, and just as effectively, as speed cameras or seeing a police car in your driving mirror deter speeding. You don't have to be arrested, or to experience the disulfiram–Alcohol Reaction, to be deterred, though either experience is reinforcing. In behavioural terms, disulfiram can also be viewed as an antagonist or 'response-preventer' but just as importantly, it facilitates exposure to cues and situations that normally lead to drinking. It does this by making it easy—or at any rate, much easier—for patients to lead an ordinary life, which means exposing themselves to ordinary drink-related cues, without actually drinking alcohol. This process has been compared to the rapid learning of a foreign language when circumstances deprive you of people who speak your usual one—a situation which any good language school will create for you in an 'immersion' course [11].
7. Patient motivation is a key factor in the success of disulfiram as a therapy. Like all drugs, disulfiram does not work if it is not taken. Many patents with alcohol dependence are very ambivalent about giving up alcohol, even for brief periods

and it follows very naturally that they are equally ambivalent about taking a drug like disulfiram which would effectively prevent them from drinking. When the mechanism of action of disulfiram is explained to patients, it is mentioned that disulfiram would help you resist temptation and prevent drinking it is often not consumed. Motivated patients that take disulfiram regularly on their own initiative are usually a type of compliant patients who would do well with any kind of treatment [12].

8. Disulfiram is a comparatively long-acting drug. Its main action is to inhibit acetaldehyde dehyrogenase (ALDH) leading to much higher levels of acetaldehyde than are normally present during drinking. This causes the facial flushing, throbbing headache, nausea and sometimes vomiting which characterizes the disulfiram–ethanol reaction. Genetically determined ALDH deficiency is common in Japan and protects against alcohol abuse. In homozygotes for the condition, alcohol abuse is apparently never seen [13]. The alcohol-sensitizing effect continues not just when disulfiram remains in blood but until new ALDH is produced. The process can take anything up to a week or more. Thus, the advantage of disulfiram is that one does not need daily administration unlike naltrexone and acamprosate. Thrice or even twice weekly dosage may be adequate [14].
9. Some clinicians believe that disulfiram is a form of punishment or aversion therapy. Aversion therapy has no place in the modern day treatment of alcohol dependence and was based on the principle is that you repeatedly combine the rehearsal of some particular undesired thought or behaviour like drinking alcohol or with an unpleasant stimulus and in this case making patients drink while taking disulfiram until they feel ill with the disulfiram–ethanol reaction. In its early days, disulfiram was used a part of aversion treatment, but it has never been used this way in the last three decades definitely [15].
10. Improving the compliance of disulfiram is a major mechanism by which its efficacy shall act. When this happens with antipsychotics in schizophrenia, we try means like depot injections. Disulfiram implants have not been very successful and there is also a fear of enhanced reactions [16]. In some cases, we try to find a formulation which only requires daily or weekly dosing rather than three or four times daily. It is imperative that we involve some third party like a family member or a community nurse and seeing that the medication is actually taken. This is routine with the very young and the very old and it ought to be routine with disulfiram and it has been proven that supervised disulfiram therapy by a caregiver or family member works best with the drug [17]. The supervisor can be a family member, provided that this is agreed beforehand and that it is also agreed that the family member can report any non-compliance to whoever is in charge of treatment. This greatly increases the incentive to comply. However, disulfiram can also be supervised during attendance at outpatient clinics, by hostel staff in the case of alcohol-dependent patients living in hostels or rehabilitation centers or by community nurses.

8.3 Surreptitious Use of Disulfiram

Disulfiram is used in a surreptitious manner at times by relatives when they want their family member to quit alcohol, but this also has been a matter of concern [18]. Many wives of alcohol-dependent patients give disulfiram to their husbands without their knowledge and precipitate a disulfiram–ethanol reaction in them. Usually, the distraught family members of alcohol-dependent patients may approach a psychiatrist in the patient's absence. Disulfiram, commonly referred to as reaction causing medicine is then given to the patient surreptitiously mixed with food or fluids. The patient starts to have a reaction after consuming alcohol and quits alcohol thinking that it is bad for him as it reacts with his body. Some clinicians believe that giving disulfiram in such a manner may possibly help some alcohol-dependent patients, especially those who are poorly motivated to quit drinking. There are chances that the patient may drink more to numb the discomforting disulfiram–ethanol reaction symptoms and may cause a more severe reaction and cause a near fatal outcome. Thus, such administration done with the hope of helping may cause harm to the patient [19]. It is interesting that in some quarters in India, god men and fakirs give disulfiram as a powder to the relatives and tell them that it is a blessed powder invoked from God to help ease their suffering and help the patient quit alcohol (personal clinical experience).

Such surreptitious administration of disulfiram raises a few ethical questions. Could prescribing in such a manner be considered ethical, especially when the patient is always too inebriated or unmotivated to co-operate with treatment. From a utilitarian perspective, the ends justify the means, i.e. since surreptitious administering of disulfiram helps in quitting alcohol, it serves the purpose and is justified. From a Kantian (deontological) perspective, some forms of conduct are obligatory irrespective of the consequences. Under such principles, stealthy efforts to help patients in potentially dangerous ways are better avoided, so that faith in the medical profession is maintained. Following the four tenets of medical ethics, prescribing disulfiram to unwitting patients severely compromises the autonomy of the patient [20].

We may sometimes have patients with psychiatric disorders like schizophrenia that are admitted against their will to prevent harm to themselves and others. The treating doctor may act in a beneficent and non-maleficent manner, but not according the patient's wishes. Following similar logic, should perpetually inebriated patients be afforded 'help' at least temporarily, especially when they harm others (recurrent fights, drunken driving) or themselves (drinking despite having liver impairment and other physical complications) [21]. Such use of disulfiram as a form coercion may lead to subsequent distrust and resentment towards doctors and undermine the efforts of the medical profession. It seems a better option to assess the capacity of the patients to consent prior to disulfiram or not administer it altogether if capacity is impaired. There is also a need for drug laws and proper training of pharmacists to regulate supply and prevent administration of disulfiram to relatives over the counter [22].

8.4 Why Is Disulfiram Under-Prescribed and Why Does It Face Opposition

There are various reasons why despite easy availability, disulfiram is underused and not a preferred line of treatment for the management of alcohol dependence. Some of them are as follows:

1. Simple ignorance of the literature available on disulfiram and its efficacy is the main one. Many researchers that are aware keep spouting the canard that controlled trials show no benefit with the drug while many studies with its success exist [22]. Some clinicians accept the evidence that supervised administration is the key to success but object that supervision can cause arguments while it may go a long way in reducing episodes of alcohol intoxication-induced domestic violence.
2. The uncalled fear of side effects is another reason. The disulfiram–alcohol reaction can be severe but actual fatalities seem to be rare. Many potential prescribers seem to believe that disulfiram is a hepatotoxic drug which must not be used in alcohol-dependent patients that have deranged livers. In reality, disulfiram-induced hepatitis occurs about once in 25,000 patient years (in my personal clinical experience not seen a case in 15 years of prescribing). Rashes are uncommon and mostly due to the activation of nickel dermatitis. Neuropathy is seen occasionally but is dose-related and nearly always reversible, especially if detected early. Patients should be informed of possible side effects and warned to report possible adverse reactions promptly [23].
3. Disulfiram is a very under-propagated drug in India. The reason is it is an old drug and companies assume that doctors are aware of it. It is also cheaper than naltrexone, acamprosate and topiramate (in India unlike the west) thereby not giving the companies as much profits and money as the other drugs (personal clinical experience).
4. Many drug prescriptions depend on ideology. The training that clinicians receive in post-graduation is what determines their prescribing practices in private practice. Many departments and deaddiction units have cultivated an environment that disulfiram is a toxic drug and must not be used and this leads to a lot of resentment being fed into the blank slate minds of post-graduate doctors about the drug. Thus they develop primitive fears that they never overcome and thus underuse the drug in their practice as well (personal clinical experience).
5. Many clinicians sadly believe that one must be motivated to give up alcohol and that drugs which can help alcoholics to drink less or abstain is not a solution and rather some kind of existential or ‘spiritual’ renaissance which will entirely change their attitude to alcohol and to life works better. For such doctors, Alcoholic Anonymous groups are the best but often the only treatment. Thus, disulfiram though useful remains under prescribed [24]. Many psychologists, therapists and social workers usually know nothing of other psychological approaches to alcoholism, let alone medical ones. Indeed, they are often hostile to disulfiram and other drugs because it means letting the doctors into their patch. Disulfiram is an out-patient treatment par excellence but underused.

6. The resistance to the deterrence model of treatment may be only one aspect of a more general trend that regards deterrence as inferior to 'positive reinforcement' (i.e. reward) in programs for changing undesirable behaviour. This position may be politically correct but is not always scientifically correct. Therapeutic strategies based on positive reinforcement principles, such as voucher-based contingency management, are relatively popular, though only modestly effective in practice. Even with escalating rewards, they can generate periods of abstinence only for as long as the incentive is provided. We emphasize that long-term supervised disulfiram aims at and optimizes the acquisition by patients of new and useful coping skills, information, insights and responses that become increasingly automatic [25].
7. Another advantage of disulfiram which is not taken advantage of is that it can be prescribed together with acamprosate or naltrexone and certainly seems to improve the effectiveness of these drugs. More importantly, it can be added to methadone mixture when alcohol abuse threatens to sabotage methadone maintenance treatment, the reduction in drinking being both significant and striking [26]. Thus, it can prevent alcohol use which may be a gateway drug and cause further relapse in multiple substance users.
8. Though allegedly unpopular with patients, supervised disulfiram is accepted by 95% of alcohol-dependent patients who had relapsed multiple times in the past [27]. It may give such patients their first experience of a significant period of abstinence, during which other psychosocial and psychological treatments can be more effectively deployed [28].

8.5 Technique of Effective Supervised Disulfiram Therapy

The involvement of a third party in supervising oral disulfiram provides additional opportunities for involving family members in the broader therapeutic and monitoring enterprise. Any failure of compliance is thus more likely to be detected and reported promptly enough for professionals to intervene, either before drinking resumes or before a mere lapse turns into a full-blown relapse [29]. An awareness of this potent combination of pharmacology, symbolism and external control and monitoring is crucial to maximizing the benefits of supervised disulfiram.

The methods for effective supervised disulfiram therapy include the following [30]:

1. Identify a disulfiram monitor who would be substantially and negatively affected by resumption of drinking, e.g. spouse, family member, employer, partner, landlord.
2. The monitor should normally have regular, ideally daily, contact with the patient.
3. Specify precisely the time and place where disulfiram could be taken conveniently, with both persons present.

4. Have disulfiram taken at a time when other forms of medication are normally taken, i.e. the 'response-chaining' principle.
5. Grind up the disulfiram tablet and dissolve it in a drink (coffee, tea, juice) to avoid any suspicion of later expulsion or check the mouth in all corners after administering the drug.
6. If the monitor is not present when the patient has taken disulfiram, the patient should take another tablet the same day, when the monitor is present, to provide absolute assurance to the monitor.
7. The patient should thank the monitor for taking the time to observe.
8. The monitor should comment on some positive attribute of the patient, that is associated with sobriety, i.e. job status, love by children, doing jobs around the house, financial security.
9. At each therapeutic session, the monitor attends with the patient, if possible, so that the therapist can instruct, supervise and provide feedback to both.
10. At each therapeutic session, disulfiram is taken in the presence of the therapist.
11. The monitor is to telephone the therapist if the patient omits taking disulfiram for 3 days; the therapist then telephones the patient to arrange a session.
12. When the usual 30-day supply of tablets is nearly depleted, the monitor prompts and assists the patient to renew the prescription; failure to do so has been one of the most apparent major causes of discontinuing disulfiram.
13. The therapist asks the patient and monitor to rehearse probable situations which cause the reluctance to take the disulfiram, and teaches them how to overcome such interferences.
14. The patient is taught to view the use and ritual of taking disulfiram as a means of providing assurance to themselves and their loved ones that they will not succumb to temptations that are otherwise beyond their control.
15. It is emphasized that the central feature is the patient's desire, not coercion.

8.6 Conclusions

Disulfiram has been in use for the past six decades and has had its fair share of proponents and detractors. The use of disulfiram is a story skewed with faith, lack of literacy and at times, false beliefs imposed on clinicians. There may be a shortage of randomized double-blind controlled trials when it comes to using disulfiram compared to other drugs in the long-term management of alcohol dependence. No one asks for controlled studies when it comes to administering saline in dehydration or glucose in hypoglycemia. Similarly, clinicians that use disulfiram have a certain amount of blind faith in the molecule propelled by the success seen with it. While disulfiram may have its rivals, its important not to underplay the change in lives for hundreds of families that it has brought about by one member being prevented from consuming alcohol. Disulfiram as a treatment is here to stay and its death nowhere in site for years to come.

References

1. Suh JJ, Pettinati HM, Kampman KM, O'Brien CP. The status of disulfiram: a half of a century later. J Clin Psychopharmacol. 2006;26(3):290–302.
2. Savas MC, Güllü İH. Disulfiram–ethanol test reaction: significance of supervision. Ann Pharmacother. 1997;31(3):374–5.
3. Brewer C, Meyers RJ, Johnsen J. Does disulfiram help to prevent relapse in alcohol abuse ? CNS Drugs. 2000;14(5):329–41.
4. Lima MS, Soares BG, Reisser AA, Farrell M. Pharmacological treatment of cocaine dependence: a systematic review. Addiction. 2002;97(8):931–49.
5. Chick J. Safety issues concerning the use of disulfiram in treating alcohol dependence. Drug Saf. 1999;20(5):427–35.
6. Brewer C. Long-term, high-dose disulfiram in the treatment of alcohol abuse. Br J Psychiatry. 1993;163(5):687–9.
7. Jørgensen CH, Pedersen B, Tønnesen H. The efficacy of disulfiram for the treatment of alcohol use disorder. Alcohol Clin Exp Res. 2011;35(10):1749–58.
8. Agosti V. The efficacy of treatments in reducing alcohol consumption: a meta-analysis. Int J Addict. 1995;30(8):1067–77.
9. Skinner MD, Lahmek P, Pham H, Aubin HJ. Disulfiram efficacy in the treatment of alcohol dependence: a meta-analysis. PLoS One. 2014;9(2):e87366.
10. Dolan SL, Rohsenow DJ, Martin RA, Monti PM. Urge-specific and lifestyle coping strategies of alcoholics: relationships of specific strategies to treatment outcome. Drug Alcohol Depend. 2013;128(1–2):8–14.
11. Brewer C, Streel E. Learning the language of abstinence in addiction treatment: some similarities between relapse-prevention with disulfiram, naltrexone, and other pharmacological antagonists and intensive "immersion" methods of foreign language teaching. Subst Abuse. 2003;24(3):157–73.
12. Brewer C. On the specific effectiveness, and under-valuing, of pharmacological treatments for addiction: a comparison of methadone, naltrexone and disulfiram with psychosocial interventions. Addict Res. 1996;3(4):297–313.
13. Harada S, Agarwal DP, Goedde HW, Ishikawa B. Aldehyde dehydrogenase isozyme variation and alcoholism in Japan. Pharmacol Biochem Behav. 1983;18:151–3.
14. Krampe H, Spies CD, Ehrenreich H. Supervised disulfiram in the treatment of alcohol use disorder: a commentary. Alcohol Clin Exp Res. 2011;35(10):1732–6.
15. Fuller RK, Gordis E. Does disulfiram have a role in alcoholism treatment today? Addiction. 2004;99(1):21–4.
16. Hughes JC, Cook CC. The efficacy of disulfiram: a review of outcome studies. Addiction. 1997;92(4):381–95.
17. Krampe H, Ehrenreich H. Supervised disulfiram as adjunct to psychotherapy in alcoholism treatment. Curr Pharm Des. 2010;16(19):2076–90.
18. Sarkar S. Surreptitious use of disulfiram. Indian J Med Ethics. 2013;10:71–2.
19. Manjunatha N, Vidyendaran R, Rao MG, Kulkarni GB, Muralidharan K, John JP, Amar BR, Jain S. Subacute vocal cord paralysis, facial palsy and paraesthesias of lower limbs following surreptitious administration of disulfiram. J Neurol Neurosurg Psychiatry. 2010;81(12):1409–10.
20. Mangot AG. Ethical aspects of surreptitious use of disulfiram. J Subs Use. 2017;22(3):244–5.
21. Alharbi FF, el-Guebaly N. The relative safety of disulfiram. Addict Disord Treat. 2013;12(3):140–7.
22. Barth KS, Malcolm RJ. Disulfiram: an old therapeutic with new applications. CNS Neurol Disord Drug Targets. 2010;9(1):5–12.
23. O'Shea B. Disulfiram revisited. Hosp Med. 2000;61(12):849–51.
24. Vaillant GE. Alcoholics anonymous: cult or cure? Austr N Z J Psychiatry. 2005;39(6):431–6.

25. Martin B, Clapp L, Bialkowski D, Bridgeford D, Amponsah A, Lyons L, Beresford TP. Compliance to supervised disulfiram therapy: a comparison of voluntary and court-ordered patients. Am J Addict. 2003;12(2):137–43.
26. Diehl A, Ulmer L, Mutschler J, Herre H, Krumm B, Croissant B, Mann K, Kiefer F. Why is disulfiram superior to acamprosate in the routine clinical setting? A retrospective long-term study in 353 alcohol-dependent patients. Alcohol Alcohol. 2010;45(3):271–7.
27. Carroll KM, Nich C, Ball SA, McCance E, Rounsavile BJ. Treatment of cocaine and alcohol dependence with psychotherapy and disulfiram. Addiction. 1998;93(5):713–27.
28. Carroll KM. Recent advances in the psychotherapy of addictive disorders. Curr Psychiatry Rep. 2005;7(5):329–36.
29. Brewer C. Patterns of compliance and evasion in treatment programmes which include supervised disulfiram. Alcohol Alcohol. 1986;21(4):385–8.
30. Azrin NH, Sisson RW, Meyers R, Godley M. Alcoholism treatment by disulfiram and community reinforcement therapy. J Behav Ther Exp Psychiatry. 1982;13(2):105–12.

MIX
Papier aus verantwortungsvollen Quellen
Paper from responsible sources
FSC® C105338

If you have any concerns about our products,
you can contact us on
ProductSafety@springernature.com

In case Publisher is established outside the EU,
the EU authorized representative is:
Springer Nature Customer Service Center GmbH
Europaplatz 3, 69115 Heidelberg, Germany

Printed by Libri Plureos GmbH
in Hamburg, Germany